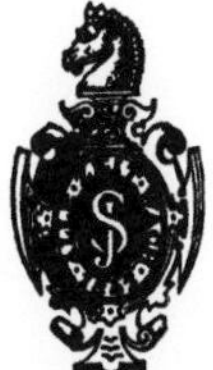

Recent Results in Cancer Research

Fortschritte der Krebsforschung

Progrès dans les recherches sur le cancer

31

Edited by

*V. G. Allfrey, New York · M. Allgöwer, Basel · K. H. Bauer, Heidelberg
I. Berenblum, Rehovoth · F. Bergel, Jersey · J. Bernard, Paris · W. Bernhard, Villejuif · N. N. Blokhin, Moskva · H. E. Bock, Tübingen · P. Bucalossi, Milano · A. V. Chaklin, Moskva · M. Chorazy, Gliwice · G. J. Cunningham, Richmond · W. Dameshek †, Boston · M. Dargent, Lyon · G. Della Porta, Milano · P. Denoix, Villejuif · R. Dulbecco, La Jolla · H. Eagle, New York
R. Eker, Oslo · P. Grabar, Paris · H. Hamperl, Bonn · R. J. C. Harris, London
E. Hecker, Heidelberg · R. Herbeuval, Nancy · J. Higginson, Lyon
W. C. Hueper, Fort Myers · H. Isliker, Lausanne · D. A. Karnofsky †, New York · J. Kieler, København · G. Klein, Stockholm · H. Koprowski, Philadelphia · L. G. Koss, New York · G. Martz, Zürich · G. Mathé, Villejuif
O. Mühlbock, Amsterdam · W. Nakahara, Tokyo · V. R. Potter, Madison
A. B. Sabin, Rehovoth · L. Sachs, Rehovoth · F. A. Saxén, Helsinki
W. Szybalski, Madison · H. Tagnon, Bruxelles · R. M. Taylor, Toronto
A. Tissières, Genève · E. Uehlinger, Zürich · R. W. Wissler, Chicago
T. Yoshida, Tokyo*

Editor in chief
P. Rentchnick, Genève

Springer-Verlag Berlin · Heidelberg · New York 1970

Pierre Denoix

Treatment of Malignant Breast Tumors

Indications and Results

*A Study Based on 1174 Cases Treated at the
Institut Gustave-Roussy between 1954 and 1962*

Translated into English by Barbara Crook

With 18 Figures

Springer-Verlag Berlin · Heidelberg · New York 1970

Professor P. Denoix, Director,
Institut Gustave-Roussy, F-94 Villejuif

Sponsored by the Swiss League against Cancer

ISBN-13: 978-3-642-99983-3   e-ISBN-13: 978-3-642-99981-9
DOI: 10.1007/978-3-642-99981-9

With Collaboration of

Medicine

Georges Brulé · Paul Juret · Jacqueline Roujeau
Françoise May-Lévin

Radiology

Paul Markovits · Danielle Sarrazin

Surgery

Jean Génin · Michel Hayem · Jean Lacour

Pathological Anatomy

Geneviève Contesso · Gabrielle Vogt-Hoerner

Statistics

Monique Lê · Claude Rouquette

Contents

Introduction

One of the chief concerns of the medical staff of the Institut Gustave-Roussy is to find the right indications for treating every cancer site, and particularly cancer of the breast. The best treatment is the one which offers the patient the best chance of recovery, yet is at the same time the simplest and least mutilating [36].

It is our policy at the Institut, rather than to lay down a series of therapeutic measures which are applied systematically to all patients, to be selective, that is, to determine the best treatment for each individual patient. We make extensive use of prognostic factors, not merely for retrospective assessment when the treatment is completed, but very early on—during treatment or even before it is begun; thus, the treatment may be changed as a result, or simplified from the outset, when it is thought the outcome will be equally satisfactory.

Our appreciation of the prognostic value of this or that clinical or biological factor is still far from complete, and we are continuing our studies in this direction. We already recognize a certain number of factors from which we try to extract the maximum information. Of these, the most important is the condition of the lymph nodes: the presence (N+) or absence (N−) of histologically confirmed lymphatic invasion. The prognostic value of such information has long been known, but it is our aim to obtain it as early as possible and then to base most of our therapeutic indications upon it. This is why we consider early histological examination of the lymph nodes so important, at least, until we find a better—by which we mean earlier—indicator.

With these ideas in mind, we have based the Institut's current treatment schedule for mammary carcinoma on a few simple principles:

1. Surgery, wherever possible, is the basic treatment.

2. This always means ablation of at least the whole breast.

3. Depending on the location of the tumor within the breast and the condition of the axillary lymph nodes, surgery is extended to include internal mammary structures.

4. Where there is invasion of the lymph nodes (N+), surgery is followed by radiotherapy.

5. Cases which are inoperable on referral receive high-dose radiotherapy. The initial extent of the lesions and their condition after irradiation are the principal criteria forming an indication for complementary surgery.

6. In pre-menopausal women, or those in whom the menopause occurred less than 2 years before, castration is done concurrently with radiotherapy on patients who were initially operable but are N+, and on all other initially inoperable patients, whether N+ or N−.

7. Combined treatments, especially surgery + radiotherapy, with or without hormone therapy, are regarded as a coherent whole and not as a sequence of separate events.

8. The treatment plan is also based on the individual features of the patient, such as age, general condition and medical history, which might furnish reasons for deviating from the basic plan.

This study is based essentially upon the 1174 patients seen at the Institut Gustave-Roussy between 1954 and 1962.

I. The Institut's Contribution to the Definition of Factors Guiding the Choice of Treatment

A. Phase of Development

The concept of "phase of development" is a relatively new one which we think highly of at the Institut Gustave-Roussy, where it was emphasized by RENÉ HUGUENIN [1]. We are endeavoring to show its importance and to define its characteristics, but it must be said in fairness that, as regards the field of carcinology in general, we were not the first to use the concept of phase of development, which evolved in the course of experimental work on cancer. It took on fresh importance in the light of recent research on the duration of the cell cycle and the "doubling time" of tumors.

The primitive malignant tumor arises initially from a modification of one or more cells at a time when conditions favor their growth. The cells multiply by successive divisions, thus creating several cell clones. These clones combine to form the initial tumor mass [62].

Let us assume for the time being that growth is possible on the basis of this clone or clones, and that all the cells formed by each successive division participate in the next. Let us also assume, to simplify the model, that the duration of the cell cycle is constant. There may be variations in its length, but it seems likely that the inability to rest may be a characteristic of malignant cells. At the experimental level there have been many investigations which permit us to say that in most cases the cycle lasts approximately 5—10 days. In order to reach a diameter of 1 cm, a tumor consisting of malignant cells alone would have to contain some 10^9 cells, representing 30 divisions. This would require 150—300 days of "hidden life", since a tumor of 1 cm diameter is generally the smallest which is clinically detectable.

In point of fact, a solid tumor composed exclusively of malignant cells is practically never found, as a tumor needs a minimum of at least one stroma in order to subsist. This occupies a certain amount of space, and it does not grow at the same rate as the malignant cells. Furthermore, all the cells resulting from a division do not necessarily participate in the next. There are several reasons for this:

1. some will not be capable of division (abortion);

2. some may not find the necessary nutrients, particularly where they are very numerous, and thus will die (necrosis);

3. some may be destroyed by a defense mechanism of the tumor-bearing host; these defense mechanisms may take several forms (destruction);

4. some will leave the tumor and, if not destroyed, cause metastases (escape).

The growth in the volume of the tumor will also be regulated by successive divisions. There is thus a doubling period which is the expression of the mean inter-

1*

nal variation of the whole tumor (malignant tissue plus stroma). Each tumor will therefore have its own rhythm of growth which is the resultant of the sum of the factors described above, the determining factor being the number of cells unable to take part in the next division. We call this the "coefficient of loss" and it is the sum of abortion, necrosis, destruction and escape.

The host-tumor reaction and its variations will modify the coefficient of loss, introducing irregularities into the growth curve. A progressive phase of development would be due to lower losses, resulting from a decline in the host's capacity for defense and expressed in an acceleration in the rate of growth. Although we postulated a cycle of constant length, we did not exclude the possibility that it might vary or decline. This, then, is yet another variable.

Stability in a tumor is the result of a coefficient of loss of about 50%, if we make allowance for the space occupied by the stroma and its own rhythm of growth. So a stable tumor may indeed be composed of actively dividing cells. If the coefficient of loss exceeds 50%, the tumor will regress; if it is 100%, this is what we call "spontaneous cure".

So far, we have considered only the spontaneous type of development. It will readily be appreciated that the object of therapeutic measures is to raise the coefficient of loss to a level where it approaches 100%.

We possess some data on human tumors. Thus, MacDonald [45] has published some estimates for malignant breast tumors. He deduced from his observations on a number of patients that tumor doubling time for this type of cancer is between 23 and 209 days. Let us state in passing that this average time varies according to whether the lymph nodes are involved or not: 128 days for forms without histological invasion of the satellite lymph nodes (N−) and 85 days for forms with invasion of the satellite lymph nodes (N+). With the shortest doubling time, i. e. 23 days, it will take two years to grow from one cell to a tumor 1 cm in diameter. As the average tumor doubling time in the series studied was 3 months, the average time taken to progress from one cell to a tumor 1 cm in diameter would be eight years. It would of course be much longer at the other extreme of 209 days.

The 1 cm diameter represents more or less the minimum size of tumor which is clinically detectable. This is a random physical fact which has nothing whatever to do with the physiopathology of the tumor. Thus, with the equipment available to us at present, we shall on average not detect a breast tumor until eight years after its true beginning. Carrying the argument still further, we can say that it will take only two more years for the tumor to reach a diameter of 2 cm. Eight years from zero to 1 cm; two years from 1 cm to 2 cm—thus, the clinical extension increases very rapidly after detection.

We mentioned that the coefficient of loss includes allowance for cells leaving the main tumor to go elsewhere, until they reach a point at which they are either accepted, or destroyed. This contributes to the decline in the initial capital, since the missing cells do not take part in subsequent cell divisions in the tumor. The groups of cells which have gone elsewhere will, unless they are destroyed, start up in their turn at the sites where they are accepted and divide according to their own rhythm. If we assume, as a working hypothesis, that cells from the same clone maintain the same rhythm wherever they go, the metastatic foci, once accepted, will reach the 1-cm level later than the primary tumor, and the difference in time will be equal to the time lapse between the transformation of the first cell giving birth to the primary tumor and the time of their acceptance in the remote organ.

It is obvious that the action of therapeutic agents will influence one growth parameter: cell loss. The Institut Gustave-Roussy [62] was among the first to show that the other growth parameters might be influenced in the opposite direction. For instance, although a certain number of cancer cells are killed by X-rays, the growth of the survivors can be seen to accelerate. This shows that a good treatment not only increases cell losses but also checks (or at least does not stimulate) the growth of the surviving cells.

Thus the rhythm of development may be modified by a number of factors; unfortunately, they seldom go as far as complete regression, but they can certainly modify the growth curve. This is why we for several years now at the Institut Gustave-Roussy have been stressing the possibility, demonstrated by L. FOULDS [8], that a carcinoma has an irregular rhythm of development, made up of stable and progressive periods. It is reasonable to suppose that these development phases correspond to variations in the host's ability to fight them.

Malignant tumors may be placed in three groups: stationary, slow-growing and fast-growing. It has been found that the survival rate for each group is constant, and is not affected by the time lag between detection and treatment. A stationary tumor is no more serious after 6 months than it was before; a fast-growing tumor is just as serious if we catch it 6 months sooner. The important difference lies in the relative severity of these three groups. The difference as between the first and last of these groups of breast tumors (Table 1) is that, when the patient is seen more than 6 months after the first symptom, 5-year survival rates are 73 and 18% respectively, while, when it is less than 6 months, they are 69 and 22.

Table 1. *Time and size relationship*

Malignant tumors of the breast	4-yr survival/speed of development				
Time lag	< 6 months		> 6 months		Signifi-cance
	No.	Survival	No.	Survival	
Tumor static	127	69%	79	73%	NS
Slow devpt	47	45%	54	31%	NS
Fast devpt	18	22%	17	18%	NS
Significance		***		***	

$p < 0.001$ *** NS = not significant

Thus, the important fact is how long a tumor takes to reach a certain size, not time or size alone. This should not surprise us, and for two reasons:

1. the time lag in seeing the patient is only one factor in the natural history of the tumor and represents but a brief period in its long life;

2. it is most probable that such serious complications as distant metastases will have set in before this arbitrary point in time.

We must therefore have the wisdom to attribute to early diagnosis a purely relative value, because at most it cannot represent more than a few months of gain in a total history of perhaps over ten years; its importance is thus trivial in proportion. This is not to say that it is unnecessary to examine a patient and institute treatment without delay, because there is always the risk of a new event occurring, but again, when we relate this risk to the total number of events which may occur in the history of the tumor, we see that the number of events likely to occur during the only period we can control is not very large.

In any case, the "developing" forms of breast cancer, evidence of a severe imbalance in host-tumor relations, should always be taken seriously, whatever form of treatment is adopted. The patterns of treatment are still open to discussion; we report here our observations on 87 "developing" cases seen at the Institut Gustave-Roussy between 1955 and 1961 [47].

Before doing so, however, I should like to define what we mean by developing forms and to explain the classification we use. They are characterized by rate of spread and speed of development, whether the phase of development is primary, coinciding with the first symptom of the cancer, or secondary, following a period of quiescence or plateau. We distinguish three stages, according to the seriousness of the clinical picture:

1. PEV 3—very severe cases, corresponding to the classic acute forms, and involving the whole of the breast which is much inflamed. The breast is red and burning with diffused dermal and subdermal edema, its appearance being described clinically as "peau d'orange". There is nearly always collateral circulation and usually one or more extensive adenopathies embedded in the edema. This is the picture generally seen in young pregnant women with mastitis carcinosa, but it can occur with certain variations outside pregnancy and even at a fairly advanced age.

2. PEV 2—cases of medium severity, corresponding to the pseudo-inflammatory acute or subacute forms, but where only part of the breast is involved. However, the pre- and peritumoral edema usually extends beyond the limits of the tumor, which are sometimes difficult to determine. The adenopathy is similar to that described in the previous category and may be connected with the tumor by an indurated strand of neoplastic lymphangitis.

3. PEV 1—the apparently least severe cases, and also the most difficult to define. They are distinguished from the usual forms of breast cancer by a single important feature: rapid growth in the volume of the tumor. Indeed, apart from mild edema, there are usually none of the classic signs of inflammation. But the criterion of rapid growth in size (at the Institut Gustave-Roussy we call any tumor which appears to have doubled in volume within 6 months "developing") depends essentially on the outcome of questioning the patient, the subjectivity of whose assessment is well known.

There are some very limited forms which are hard to classify, and this is where mammography becomes important in the examination of breast tumors in the developing phase. The advantage of this procedure is that it offers an objective approach to the diagnosis of developing forms. It may reveal a sure sign which we call the "malignant edema picture" (see Figs. 4—8, pp. 27—30); this appears in the form of a transparent area around the tumor which is simultaneously dermal, subdermal and glandular and is accompanied by a thickening of the skin. Any tumor which on the clinical evidence does not fall into categories PEV 2 and PEV 3 but which shows the mammographic signs described should be considered to be developing (PEV 1), even if it is small in size.

We wish to stress that, while there is general agreement that initial surgery is contraindicated for forms PEV 2 and PEV 3, those classed as PEV 1, which in our experience represent some 10% of the forms classically judged to be operable, are not usually considered non-surgical. For more than twenty years we have been issuing warnings that initial surgery is hazardous in such forms of breast cancer, and we have given pride of place, if not exclusive place, to radiotherapy.

In the 87 cases observed and followed up for longer than five years (1954—1962), the 5-year survival rate for all three PEV forms was 19%. For the separate categories, see Tables 2 and 3.

We shall now discuss the results in each category in detail.

Table 2. *Survival rates*

	No. of cases	5-yr survival without recurrence	
PEV 1	36	13	36%
PEV 2	27	3	11%
PEV 3	24	0	0%
Total	87	16	19%

Table 3. *Chronological sequence of deaths as a function of developing phase*

	Death occurred during year				
	1	2	3	4	5
PEV 1 (23 deaths, 36 cases)	2	5	12	3	1
PEV 2 (24 deaths, 27 cases)	6	11	1	3	3
PEV 3 (24 deaths, 24 cases)	4	9	8	3	0
	12	25	20	9	4

1. Acute Developing Growths (PEV 3)

There were 24 cases.

The symptoms were the classic ones: invasion of the entire breast with diffused clinical and radiological edema, and obvious signs of inflammation.

The average age of the patients in this group was 56; only three were under 40 (36, 38 and 39) and five were over 64. So this is not a form peculiar to young or pregnant women, as used to be said.

The time lag between the first symptom and treatment was on average 6 months.

Table 4 shows the distribution of these cases according to UICC's TNM classification (see p. 65).

It may be thought surprising that there are eight T3 cases. The explanation is simple: even tumors less than 10 cm in diameter can invade the entire mammary gland in small breasts.

Table 4. *Distribution of PEV 3 group within the T N M classification*
(all cases are MO, i. e. without distant metastases)

	T1	T2	T3	T4	Total
N0	—	—	—	—	—
N1	—	—	2	2	4
N2	—	—	4	9	13
N3	—	—	2	5	7
Total	—	—	8	16	24

In most cases an attempt was made to obtain a definite histological diagnosis on a biopsy specimen before starting treatment of any kind. But we must emphasize how difficult and uncertain this procedure is; the diffused edema often masks the true focus of the tumor, if there is one at all. The lesions are often diffused and inhomogenous and it is difficult to locate any particular focal point. This pattern reappears at the histological level, the tumor cells being irregularly diffused throughout the edematous gland. Thus, a biopsy may yield only a fragment which it is impossible to interpret. We had a case where it was repeated five times and all were negative. It can, however, be done again after the first few sessions of irradiation which sometimes have a dramatic effect on the edema and allow the carcinomatous foci to be more easily identified. Another method of obtaining histological confirmation is to do an axillary node dissection if the lymph nodes there are palpable and if two or even three biopsies have been negative.

These 24 cases classed as PEV 3 can be broken down as follows:

1. 10 cases were NX, as no lymph node was removed at the time of treatment; all were fatal.

2. 12 cases were N+ confirmed and all were fatal; average survival after the first symptom was 25 months, the shortest time being 7 months and the longest 41 months.

3. 2 cases were N— confirmed; both were fatal, the first after 31 months and the second after 34 months. It should be noted that in the second case the axillary lymph nodes had been clinically suspect but this was not confirmed; however, a histological examination of the supraclavicular lymph nodes showed them to be N+.

An analysis of this outcome shows that the first sign of active recurrence after treatment appears about 4 months after completion of post-operative irradiation. This rapid development is well known. It appears in a number of ways:

13 cases out of 24 had distant metastases marking the active relapse and responsible for the patient's death, although there was no local recurrence. Most of the metastases were in the bones (12 out of 24). They can remain isolated but, according to their situation and particularly when they are localized in the spine, they can quickly cause incidents of compression. They may be associated with other metastases and, indeed, often are.

Pleuro-pulmonary metastases were predominant in 11 cases; we also observed hepatic involvement (6 cases) and cerebral involvement (3 cases) but only one confirmed case of ovarian involvement.

These, of course, were metastases which were either clinically or surgically confirmed. Moreover, it must be recorded that all attempts to treat them, whether by irradiation or hypophysectomy, were unsuccessful. In reality, however, it is likely that infraclinical metastatic dissemination is much more widespread, as we were able to see from the findings of the only necropsy performed in this series. This patient had, in addition to clinically recognized bone lesions involving the whole of the spine, metastases of the liver and brain and invasion of the latero-aortic lymph nodes, all quite unsuspected before her death.

11 cases had local or local/regional recurrences in the form of nodules permeating the treated cutaneous area, or else in the axillary lymph nodes. In spite of high doses of radiation, there were still recurrences, in one case after 7000 rads; they occurred before the metastases in 6 cases and simultaneously in the other 5 cases.

On the whole, what the patients usually die of is a more or less generalized metastatic syndrome, although there were no local recurrences in half the cases.

2. Subacute Developing Growths (PEV 2)

We had 28 cases in this category; of these, one must be considered separately as there was a mistake in diagnosis, subsequently rectified by the histological examination, which showed the existence of a colloid epithelioma. This particular histological type often gives the clinical impression of an inflamed tumor, whereas it is in fact a relatively less serious form. The patient in question is still alive and well and shows no sign of recurrence or metastases 5 years after undergoing mastectomy following pre-operative irradiation (2500 rads). We shall therefore take into account only the 27 genuine cases.

Average age was 51.

Time from first symptom to treatment averaged $6^{1}/_{2}$ months. However, in 7 cases it exceeded one year because the growth appeared secondarily after a plateau, while in the other 20 cases the time lag was only a few months, the growth being clinically perceptible from the start.

Classification by the T N M system is shown in Table 5.

Table 5. *Distribution of PEV 2 group within the T N M classification*

	T1	T2	T3	T4	Total
N0	—	—	1	—	1
N1	—	3	12	1	16
N2	—	1	5	—	6
N3	—	—	2	2	4
Total	—	4	20	3	27

Survival as a function of lymph node invasion was as follows:

1. 8 cases NX, no lymph node being removed at the time of treatment. All were fatal.
2. 16 cases N+, 2 of whom are still alive after more than 5 years; the remaining 14 are dead, average survival time being 23 months, the shortest 3 months and the longest 60 months.
3. 3 cases N−, one of whom is still alive 5 years after treatment. The histological examination in this case was so detailed (13 lymph nodes were examined) that we were virtually certain she was N−. The second case died after 38 months and the third after 43 months; in the last case the only two lymph nodes examined were found to be negative, yet at the time of her death she had pulmonary metastases and a supraclavicular adenopathy.

It should be noted that these cases were seen at the time before we routinely examined biopsy samples of the lymph nodes; it is probable we should now have classified the last case N+.

The history of these 27 cases of PEV 2 is as follows:

metastases attacked: bones (14 cases); liver (6 cases); brain (4 cases); ovaries (1 case, discovered on castration); pleura and lungs (9 cases).

In 7 cases a local/regional occurrence was associated with metastases. These were usually permeation nodules, and only once was there a recurrence at the level of the axillary lymph nodes. The local/regional occurrence preceded the metastases in only 3 cases, while in the others, as in the PEV 3 series, they were coincident with metastases in the terminal flare-up of metastatic dissemination.

Summing up, we may say that the course of the PEV 2 series is very similar to that of PEV 3, with this fundamental difference: that 3 out of the 27 patients are cured; moreover, local/regional control seems to have been better.

3. Developing Growths (PEV 1)

The study of this group deserves special attention because, we repeat, these are forms which many authorities judge to be initially operable. We had 36 cases, all undoubtedly showing evidence of a rapid and recent increase in the volume of the tumor, but without obvious signs of inflammation. Table 6 gives their distribution according to the T N M system.

Table 6. *Distribution of PEV 1 group within the T N M classification*

	T1	T2	T3	T4	Total
N0	—	2	1	1	4
N1	—	9	17	—	26
N2	—	2	—	1	3
N3	—	1	2	—	3
Total	—	14	20	2	36

Average age of these patients on first referral was 52 years 7 months, time lag before treatment averaged 6 months.

We describe below the treatment of these 36 cases of PEV 1.

It belongs in therapeutic category B (see p. 71). Of these 36 patients:

1. 6 cases were NX, there being no confirmation of lymph node involvement at the time of treatment. Five years later, 5 are dead and one still living.

2. 19 cases N+, 3 of whom survive after 5 years. The other 16 are dead. Average survival time was 28 months, the shortest 10 months and the longest 40 months.

3. 11 cases N−, 9 of whom survive after 5 years, the other 2 dying 27 months and 30 months after the first symptom.

We can divide the cases considered in this study of developing forms into two main groups.

The first group comprises the 51 cases classed as PEV 2 and PEV 3 and includes only three 5-year survivors, all in category PEV 2. These facts bear witness to the severity of these forms and confirm the value of the criteria we have used to identify them.

The second group comprises the 36 cases classed as PEV 1, which many people do not normally think of as non-surgical. The cases in this group are considerably less serious than those in the first group, 36% having survived for over 5 years, as against 6% in the first group. On the other hand, the results are clearly less favorable than those in the non-PEV series of breast cancers, i. e. the initially operable cases, where the 5-year survival rate is 75% (see Table 36). This shows that we are right to place them in a special class, and the results confirm the validity of the criteria employed. In this group the prognostic value of the condition of the lymph nodes was particularly clear. Indeed, among the patients whose lymph nodes were examined histologically, we find three 5-year survivors among the 19 N+ and nine among the 11 N−.

B. Determining the Condition of the Lymph Nodes

The condition of the lymph nodes in the vicinity of a carcinoma is one of the best indications of the nature of the host-tumor relationship. We have long given special attention to this problem [3, 4, 38].

Anatomical-Pathological Methods of Examination

Although this section is to be devoted to matters concerning the lymph nodes, we shall first describe the various anatomical and pathological techniques of examination which, because of the information they yield, are the foundation of our treatment policy at the Institut Gustave-Roussy.

1. Macroscopic Examination and Dissection of Specimens

Biopsy specimens are taken from the breast systematically: 1. at the level of the *nipple* along the axis of the main ducts and at right angles to it; 2. at the level of the *tumor*, a section across the widest surface of each of its three spatial dimensions; 3. at the level of all *suspicious* or *initial lesions* (fibradenoma, cyst, angioma or anything suggestive of neoplastic dissemination at a distance from the tumor). These specimens are all marked up on a special form.

We consider it important to work out as precise a method as possible for revealing any lymphatic metastases in gross sections of amputated breasts, since the presence of such metastases is one of the factors determining subsequent treatment in breast cancer.

The techniques in current use at our Institute were established by Mme VOGT-HOERNER. We have for practical reasons abandoned the method of "clearing" the axillary fat with toluene (Pickren's method); we now use dissection under the magnifying glass after fixing in Bouin's solution which stains the lymph nodes bright yellow. Each lymph node is systematically located and cut into as many serial sections about 1.5 mm thick as it will yield. With the *axillary lymph nodes*, systematic calibration has enabled us to group the various nodules found either 1. according to Rouvière's anatomical scheme (however, although the central group is easy to locate, the same is not true of the external, mammary and inferior scapular groups, which are hard to differentiate), or 2. according to BERG's concept of axillary "levels" [5], formulated in 1955: the first "level" is situated outside and below the lower margin of the pectoralis minor, the second behind the posterior face of the pectoralis minor, between the upper and lower margins of the muscle, and the third above the upper margin of the pectoralis minor and comprising the subclavicular lymph nodes.

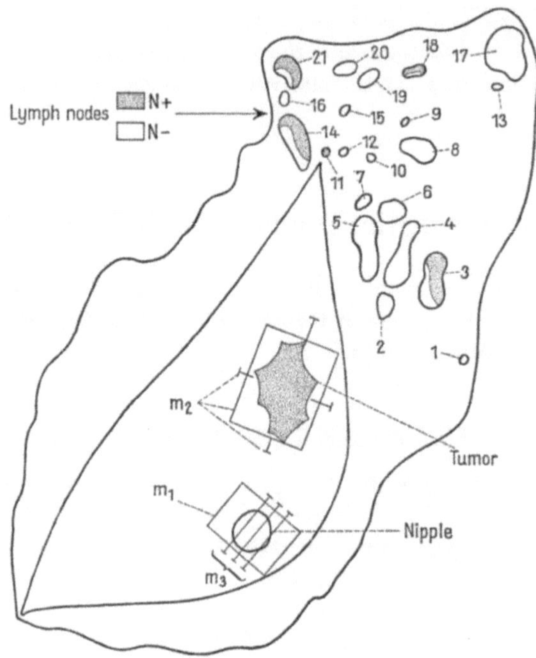

Fig. 1. *Left mastectomy with axillary dissection.* Stellate tumor of supero-external quadrant—25×25×20 mm histo-prognostic class II. Axillary lymph nodes: 5/21 N+. Madame A, age 78 years. IGR dossier No. 05/58.0159. Histology No. 55 360 (June 1958). Died June 1959

The examination of *Rotter's interpectoral lymph nodes* is always effected with great care between the two pectoral muscles, serial sections being taken across the axis of the vessels.

As regards the *internal mammary chain*, the lymph nodes are calibrated in relation to the intercostal spaces but, as the nodes in this chain are so small and extra-lymphatic metastases so common, we always carry out a symmetric serial sampling at the level of the surrounding perivascular fat.

2. Immediate Histological Examination

The gravity of the decisions which depend on their results has forced us to refine our methods. However, despite technical progress in embedding materials, we continue to use Ultropak, which some may think excessively conservative. Nevertheless, this material enables a rapid and convenient analysis to be made of large areas of tissue and with breast cancer the diagnosis often depends more on architectural than on cytological features. Here are a few examples:

the examination of *"bleeding" ducts* is done on macroscopic sections taken across the axis of the duct after rapid freezing, which gives more precise sections; *mammary cysts* are always examined on small sections taken on the periphery of the shell in the search for a small stellate carcinoma;

fibrosing-adenosis foci are diagnosed on their architectural appearance whereas, when greatly magnified, they often suggest neoplastic foci;

when *irradiated breasts* are examined with Ultropak, various zones can be analysed for vestiges of tumoral trabeculi; and finally, *axillary lymph nodes* uncovered during the operation and whose condition guides its subsequent course, can be quickly examined on the basis of several sections each, without keeping the surgeon waiting too long; some 6 to 9 are analysed as a rule before an answer is given regarding the integrity of the chain.

3. Histological Examination After Fixing and Staining

The routine procedures of histological staining with hemalum-erythrosine-saffron, in certain cases combined with a search for secretory activity in the cells by means of Mayer's mucicarmine, enable the study under the light microscope to confirm the diagnosis made during on-the-spot examination, and sometimes to upset it (in about $3^0/_0$ of cases).

The type of classification we use for the *tumor* is based on that of the WHO [1], which is set out below. The distribution of the various types of tumor among a series of cases examined in our laboratory is shown in Table 7, which follows the classification. As regards the *lymph nodes*, an exact analysis under the microscope of all the sections removed is likely to reveal the existence, not only of multiple metastases, but even of "single" metastases ($8.6^0/_0$ of axillary invasions) or "hidden" ones, in the form of a few nests of cells in the sinus bordering the lymph node (31 out of 139 N+ cases among the 518 who had Halsted's operation, that is $8.2^0/_0$). Are these perhaps cells on their way to somewhere else, or are they the first sign of metastatic invasion?

The fact that we use this technique may well explain the high incidence of N+ cases found at the Institut Gustave-Roussy: $74^0/_0$ as against $50—62^0/_0$ reported to have metastases in other published surgical series. These authors' data must therefore include some $10—20^0/_0$ of false negatives.

Classification of Breast Tumors

A. *Benign Tumors*
  1. Fibroadenoma
  2. Pure adenoma (very rare)
  3. Papillary intracanalicular cystadenoma
  4. Erosive adenomatosis of the nipple (mamillary adenoma)
  5. Benign tumors of the soft tissues: lipoma, angioma etc.

B. *Carcinomas*
  1. Non-infiltrating ductal carcinoma (strict intracanalicular adenocarcinoma)
      low papillary intraductal carcinoma;

---

[1] World Health Organization.

comedo-carcinoma;

cribriform intraductal carcinoma, or polyadenoid, or "en rognons à rosettes de Delbet"

2. Infiltrating adenocarcinoma

differentiated: tubuloacinous, papillary;

undifferentiated or atypical: trabecular, with independent cells (special form: single file);

polymorphous: the commonest type, with tubes and trabeculi combined

3. Special forms

lobular or alveolar carcinoma;

mucoid (colloid) carcinoma;

apocrine sweat gland carcinoma;

squamous-cell carcinoma (epidermoid carcinoma);

medullary carcinoma "with lymphoid infiltration" (circumscribed carcinoma);

Paget's disease of the nipple

C. *Sarcomas*

1. Derivative of a phyllode fibroadenoma

2. Other soft-tissue forms:

angiosarcoma

liposarcoma

3. (on its own) lympho- and reticulosarcoma

D. *Phyllode Tumors* (artificially isolated)

1. Fibroadenoma phyllodes

2. Cytosarcoma phyllodes, or degenerate, or fibrosarcoma.

Table 7. *Frequency of histological types of mammary carcinoma*
(437 mastectomy surgical specimens)

Histological type	No.	%
Carcinomatous cells	2	0.4
Strict intracanalicular adenocarcinoma (non-infiltrating)	2	0.4
Differentiated glanduliform adenocarcinoma (infiltrating)	52	11.3
Atypical or undifferentiated adenocarcinoma	73	16.7
Polymorphous infiltrating adenocarcinoma (combining several differentiated and undifferentiated types)	257	58.8
Lobular carcinoma (lobular or alveolar)	28	6.6
Colloid carcinoma	2	0.4
Apocrine sweat gland carcinoma	5	1.1
Medullary carcinoma	13	3.0
Other	1	

Results Obtained from a Study of the Lymph Nodes [49]

To chart the advance of metastases within the axillary lymph system, we adopted BERG's three-level notation [5] because 1. it is logical and easy to calibrate on a monobloc radical amputation; 2. it is sometimes difficult with a fixed specimen, apart from the vascular calibrations, to tell whether a lymph node belongs to the external, scapular, mammary chain, to the central group or to the axillary venous group.

Level of Invasion

The 518 cases studied [49] were grouped according to the number of axillary lymph nodes invaded, thus:

one lymph node 1 N+, two lymph nodes 2 N+ and so on. The aim was to trace the propagation of metastases in the axillary region. The results of this study are given in Table 8 under BERG's "levels" and the number of axillary metastatic localizations from 1 N+ to 10 N+.

Table 8. *Localization by level of axillary metastases in breast cancer (in the 274 cases where this information was available)*

No. of N+ lymph nodes	level 1	level 2	level 3	No. of cases (274)
1 N+	82	—	—	82
2 N+	111	8	1	60
3 N+	107	9	1	39
4 N+	113	11	—	31
5—6 N+	162	22	3	35
7—10 N+	168	41	9	27

This table shows the ascending progression of metastases from a threshold of one lymph node. It also shows that we have never had a case with second or third-level invasion without a localization at the first level. BERG's own data included one case out of 324 with third-level invasion and no localization in the other two levels. We can deduce from these results that if it were technically possible to examine without difficulty the sub-pectoral group (i. e. those situated below rather than behind the pectoralis minor), and if we could make a direct histological examination with complete and reliable results, we should find there was no invasion in the superjacent axillary nodes if there was none in this inferior group. This is a very important concept and one that can be a useful guide to the surgeon in deciding how far he should go.

Carrying precision still further in our studies, we have found that the ascending axillary invasion was very soon matched by metastases in ROTTER's interpectoral lymph nodes. Our findings are given in Table 9. In the construction of Table 8 we were unable to use all the metastatic cases because the axillary fat was not always correctly orientated, but we were able to include them all when assessing the invasion of the interpectoral lymph nodes. This explains the discrepancy between the two groups.

Table 9 shows four cases which are axillary N— and ROTTER's N+; these were cases with central or internal tumors.

This was a systematic study of the interpectoral relay stages and the 140 cases with ROTTER N— indicate that no invaded lymph nodes were found in these cases.

Table 9. *Condition of Rotter's interpectoral lymph nodes in relation to quantitative invasion of axillary lymph nodes*

No. of N+ axillary lymph nodes	Rotter N+	Rotter N−	Without Rotter	Total no. of cases
0	4			4
1	5	38	39	82
2	10	26	33	69
3		19	20	39
4	6	7	20	33
5—6	7	14	18	39
7—10	7	16	16	39
10 or more	17	20	18	65
Total	56 [a]	140	174	370

[a] The 56 Rotter N+ cases include 5 where no lymph nodes were found but where there were metastases in the interpectoral fat.

The 174 cases "without ROTTER" are cases where, despite the studies and sampling carried out, no lymph nodes at all were found. Invasion of the interpectoral chain was by no means negligible, as it was found in 11% of the 518 cases, but it was not as frequent as ROTTER supposed when he estimated that it occurred in 33% of cases.

Thus, this study enabled us to verify the progressive ascending invasion of the axillary lymph nodes in 518 cases of breast cancer. It has been asserted in the past that the axillary lymph nodes were not invaded continuously but that some stages were leapfrogged; however, this was really due to the inadequacy of the examination techniques used.

Of course, not everyone has the facilities we have for such painstaking examinations. But this very fact implies that, where they cannot be carried out, it is always wise to suspect undetected cases of N+ and to act accordingly.

In conclusion, it may be said that if it is possible to carry out a detailed and correctly orientated histological examination of the axillary surgical specimen, and the lower axillary group of lymph nodes is N−, one can reasonably conclude that there is no invasion of higher levels.

We should like to mention that at the Institut Gustave-Roussy we have never undertaken a systematic radiological exploration of the axillary or internal mammary lymph nodes by means of lymphography for fear of blurring the histological picture, although other hospitals have attempted it. It can be instructive, provided that the evidence obtained indicates where the tumor is localized.

Predicting the Condition of the Internal Mammary Chain [49]

The longer one studies the behavior of the lymphatic system in cancer in general and in malignant breast cancer in particular, the more one appreciates its importance and the more one realizes how desirable it is not to interfere surgically with a lymph-node region which has not been invaded.

Unfortunately, in the present state of the art, and indeed in most cases, we should have to cut out a lymph-node region and examine it before being able to conclude that it should not have been removed. What we need, therefore, are indirect techniques to enable us to predict the condition of the lymph nodes *in situ*.

As regards breast tumors, there is already one possibility of prediction which we have just explained: once the complete absence of invasion in the lower group of axillary lymph nodes has been reliably established, we can predict that there will be no invasion of the superjacent group. In the case of malignant breast tumors, we have a second possibility of prediction. A study of the various published works comparing the axillary and internal mammary invasion in malignant breast tumors is instructive so long as—and this not always the case—the documents presented state the localization of the tumor within the breast and give the N state of the axillary and internal mammary lymph nodes for each site. Where this is done, it will always be found that when the tumor is located in the outer quadrants of the breast, and the axillary lymph nodes have been examined by a detailed and careful technique like that used at the Institut Gustave-Roussy (see Table 10) and found to be N−, then one can predict that there is no invasion of the internal mammary lymph nodes. This concept must be borne in mind, because it is an important justification of some of the methods of treatment in use at the Institut Gustave-Roussy.

Table 10. *Local/regional invasion of lymph nodes by site of tumor*

Tumor site		UO	LO	LI	sub-mammary crease	UI	1/2 sup.	1/2 inf.	1/2 ext.	1/2 int.	whole breast	Total
Lymph nodes												
Ax.	I. M.											
N−	N−	16	3	6	1	47	16	7		2	13	111
N−	N+				2	7	3				1	13
N+	N−	92	12	5	4	32	42	3	11	3	34	238
N+	N+	39	7	4	4	24	22	5	3	3	27	138
Total		147	22	15	11	110	83	15	14	8	75	500
% Invasion of internal mammary chain		26.4	31.8	(26.6)	(54.5)	28.7	30	(33.3)	(21.4)	(37.5)	37.5	30.2

Quadrants — UO upper outer, LO lower outer, UI upper inner, LI lower inner, Ax axillary and I.M. internal mammary lymph nodes.

Note: Whenever the axillary lymph nodes were N− and the tumor was located in one of the external quadrants or straddled both external quadrants (this was the case in 111+13 =124 cases in our series of 500), there was no invasion of the internal mammary chain.

C. Recurrence and Invasion of Lymph Nodes

A special study has been carried out to try to identify the later "developing" manifestations of malignant breast tumors according to whether the patient was N− or N+ at the time of the first treatment. This is a fairly old study [4] and the analytical techniques used are open to criticism; moreover, the lymph nodes were not examined with the precision that Mme VOGT-HOERNER has since introduced. Nevertheless, it will be seen that the conclusions drawn from this study have been consistently confirmed by subsequent findings.

The study covered 278 cases whose axillary lymph nodes had been histologically examined. The position after 5 years was as follows: of the 161 N— cases, 110 were still living and 51 were dead; of the 117 N+ cases, 51 were living and 66 dead. Thus among the 278 patients there were 117 deaths within 5 years or, to put it another way, there was a 58% survival. Classified by N state, N— showed a 68% survival (51 deaths among 161 patients) and N+ a 44% survival (66 deaths among 117 patients).

The difference in the survival rates certainly shows that there is a disparity between the N— and N+ groups, the probability of finding such a distribution by chance being only one in a thousand. Thus we are justified in saying that the 5-year survival rate shows a significant difference between the two groups.

The numbers of N— and N+ being 161 and 117 respectively, 42% of these 278 cases were N+. The type of treatment given was not included within the terms of reference of this study, so that we cannot comment on this. However, we can say that we have confirmed that no distinction was made in the type of treatment administered to the two groups. To give meaning to a comparison between the groups studied, the following method was applied: the two groups to be studied were N— deceased (51 cases) and N+ deceased (66 cases). The groups were levelled down to 51 to match the size of the smaller group. The 15 cases taken out of the N+ group were those with case numbers farthest from those of the N— group; the elimination was done on the basis of the numbers alone, the medical history of the patients being unknown to the person making the selection.

All 117 patients were followed up; unfortunately, for 24, though the date of death is known, the manner of it is not known. However, as these 24 were evenly distributed between the 2 groups, we may take it that the result is not affected by this lack of information. There were 13 deaths attributed to intercurrent illness among the N— group, therefore 13 cases with numbers closest to these were taken out of the N+ group, leaving 26 comparable cases in each group.

Table 11 gives the main clinical findings attributable to cancer found in the two series. A comparison of the relative frequency of the 4 possible sites included shows a distinct difference between the two groups. The forms with lymph node invasion (N+) are manifested in local/regional lesions (15 cases), whereas this is exceptional

Table 11. *Main secondary deposit related to death*

Group	Bone metastases	Disseminated metastases	Pulmonary metastases	Local/regional recurrences
N—	15	8	7	2 (both with bone metastases)
N+	4	2	7	15 (2 of these had pulmonary metastases and 2 disseminated metastases)

Note: Sites quoted are those recorded in the case notes; they do not exclude the possibility of other associated but unidentified localizations. These therefore are the clinically predominant manifestations. In several cases, more than one were found in the same patient.

in the N− group (2 cases). These local/regional lesions comprise thoracic and cutaneous nodules as well as axillary and supra-clavicular adenopathies.

This difference in frequency is reversed for bone metastases: 15 cases N−, as against 4 N+; moreover, if we add the disseminated cases without definite sites in the bone, we get 23 N− and 6 N+.

A study of Fig. 2 raises three questions concerning the respective significance of new manifestations. Pulmonary metastases were omitted because the same number occurred in each group.

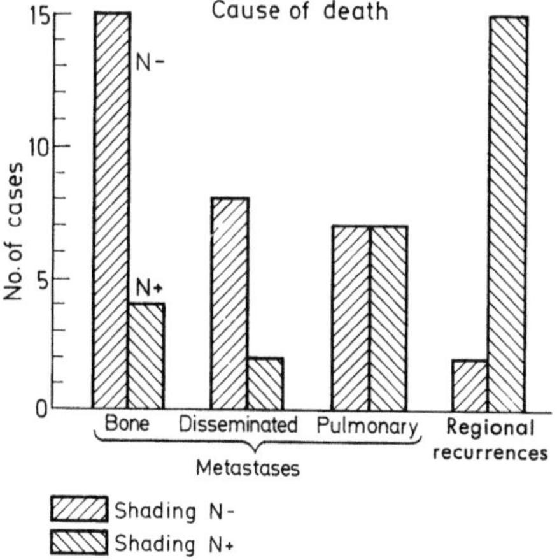

Fig. 2. *Main secondary deposit related to death*

1. Bone Metastases

We may ask whether the fact that 15 cases were found in the N− group and 4 in the N+ is random and can be attributed to chance. A statistical analysis shows that the probability of obtaining such figures by chance is 1.5 per thousand. So we are justified in assuming that there is a significant and non-random difference in the frequency of bone metastases in the two groups.

2. Disseminated Metastases

We may ask the same question concerning disseminated metastases, which occur 4 times as often in the N− group. Here the probability of this being due to chance is 3%, so we may suppose that the distribution is not random.

3. Local/regional Recurrences

Similar calculations give a probability of 1 in 10,000 of finding such a distribution by chance. We may therefore assume it is not random.

A statistical analysis of these facts shows that they are unquestionably not due to chance and that the probability of their occurring is very slight, being between 3% and 1 in 10,000. We are therefore justified in assuming that there is a formal link between the number of recurrences or metastases and the N− and N+ groups of cancers examined. In view of these distinct differences, it is remarkable that the frequency of pulmonary metastases (7 : 7) is the same.

The N− forms are not subject to local/regional dissemination, the failures here being due to distant metastases which were not influenced by local treatment. It became clear to us in the course of this study that there is little likelihood of local recurrence in the N− forms. What we have learned since about the need for precision in the N examination has brought home to us that at the time this study was made (some years ago, it will be recalled), some N+ cases were still being classed as N−. We have therefore accepted the hypothesis that among the true N− cases, where no doubts persist about the state of the lymph nodes, there should in general be no further local/regional manifestations.

We shall see that so far this hypothesis remains unshaken.

D. Metastases of Breast Cancers

We thought there would be some value in studying breast cancer via the anatomical checks which are carried out systematically at the Institut Gustave-Roussy. The following analysis [64] comprises 114 breast cancer patients on whom an autopsy was carried out during the period January 1960 to January 1966, representing 10% of the total of all confirmed localizations during this period (1103 cases) and 4% of

Table 12. *Metastatic dissemination in 114 breast cancer patients (confirmed at necropsy)*

Visceral metastases	No.	%	Lymph-node metastases	%
Above diaphragm			*Above diaphragm*	
Broncho-pulmonary	66	57	Mediastinal	31
Pleural	44	39	Intertracheal bronchial	12
Cutaneous	27	24	Cervical	6
Heart	18	16	Pretracheal	4
Thyroid	17	15		
Esophagus	2	2		
Larynx	1	1		
Below diaphragm			*Below diaphragm*	
Liver	76	67	Aortic	24
Adrenals	35	31	Lumbar	20
Ovaries	20	18	Pancreatic	9.8
Kidney	16	14	Iliac	5
Uterus	12	11	Inguinal	1
Spleen	11	10	Hepatic	1
Pancreas	10	9		
Stomach	4	4		
Intestine	3	3		
Ureter	3	3		
Rectum	2	2		
Bladder	2	2		
Vagina	2	2		
Vertebral	80	70		

Note: M0 7 cases without metastases (6%). M+ 107 cases with metastases (94%).

the patients referred to the Institut for breast cancer (2930 patients) during this period.

This is, of course, a "biased" population, particularly in the matter of the treatment of mammary carcinomas, because of the techniques of hypophysectomy practised at the Institut for extensive cancers, but this represents only a small proportion of all patients. Concerning the others, we might ask, in view of the fact that it tends to be social and economic or psychological factors rather than any particular feature of the disease which determine whether patients spend the terminal phase of cancer in hospital, whether our series does not after all give a fair reflection of the dissemination caused by tumors throughout the body, qualitatively speaking, at any rate.

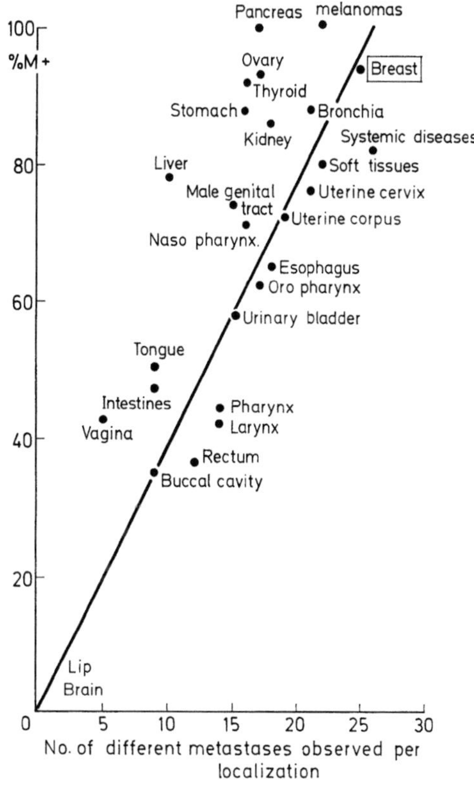

Fig. 3. *Metastatic dissemination of cancers of all origins* (based on 1103 necropsies in the period 1960—1966)

Owing to the technique used, Table 12 does not include bone metastases other than those of the vertebrae.

This series, which is comparable with those published by other authors, shows on the one hand the importance of bone metastases (70%), metastases of the liver (68%) and pleuro-pulmonary and mediastinal lymph-node disseminations, which are usually identified clinically or by X-rays, and on the other hand the sub-diaphragmatic invasion extending to the lumbar-aortic and iliac chains as well as to the adrenals (35 cases out of 107), the latter apparently having a silent development. We should perhaps make the examinations designed to detect them more systematic and, with the insight this will give us, introduce new therapeutic measures.

Finally, if we compare the metastatic dissemination of breast cancers with that of other tumor localizations, we see from Fig. 3, based on the 1103 autopsies done at the Institut Gustave-Roussy, that the "likelihood of metastases" with breast cancer is one of the highest in our series.

E. Other Factors Having Prognostic Value and Providing Criteria for the Orientation of Therapy
[14, 15, 26, 27, 28, 29, 35, 58]

1. How to use the Idea of Prognosis

Prognosis means "foreknowledge" [2] and its study consists in predicting future events on the basis of present happenings. Applying this definition to the study of cancer, we can envisage the possibility of a series of predictions corresponding to the successive stages of development of the cancer. These stages may be expressed schematically as follows:

1. detection of cancer and evolution before first treatment;
2. balance sheet immediately before first treatment;
3. first treatment and balance sheet during course of therapy;
4. apparent cure;
5. stabilization;
6. new manifestation: balance sheet and therapy.

2. Histological Grading of Breast Carcinomas for Prognostic Purposes

Already in the 19th century pathologists were trying to break out of the rigid framework of morphological description of breast cancer and to regroup certain factors concerning the tissues which could be interpreted as allowing prognosis; they were seeking a relationship between the degree of anaplasia or lack of morphological differentiation of mammary tumors relative to the cells from which they derive, and the survival of the patient.

Having used GRICOUROFF's grading for a number of years, we changed over in 1962 to that proposed by SCARFF and taken up again by BLOOM and RICHARDSON [24], as we considered it more objective (Table 13).

There are 3 criteria: degree of differentiation of the tumor, its nuclear pleomorphism, and the mitotic activity or hyperchromatism of its nuclei. Each is scored from 1 to 3 and, according to the total number of points, the tumor under study is placed in one of three grades of increasing malignity:

Grade I   — 3—5 points, prognosis favorable;
Grade II — 6—7 points, prognosis slightly worse;
Grade III — 8 or 9 points, prognosis poor.

---

[2] To predict that treatment will be unsuccessful and then see the patient cured is proof that the prediction was wrong, i. e. it was a "bad prognosis".

Table 13. *Histological grading of mammary cancers (Method of* SCARFF *and* BLOOM)

Grade given	I	II	III
Criterion observed			
Degree of differentiation	Glanduliform cavities all over	Cavities combined with trabeculi	No glanduliform cavities at all
Degree of nuclear pleomorphism	All nuclei regular	Moderate irregularities	Very many malformed nuclei
Mitotic activity or nuclear hyperchromatism	Max. 1 mitosis per field	2 mitoses per field	At least 3 mitoses per field

(magnification: ×250)

Table 14. *Distribution of cases by T N M classification with survival rates*

| Grade | T1 | | T2 | | T3 | | Unknown | Total | 5-yr survival | |
	N−	N+	N−	N+	N−	N+			No. of cases living	% survival
I	4	3	21	31	—	2	1	62	59	95
II	6	9	19	56	—	7	1	98	77	79
III	8	8	12	44	—	—	1	73	31	42
Total	18	20	53	131	—	9	3	233	167	72

Table 15. *Histo-prognostic classification. Lymph-node metastases and survival*

Grade		Alive after 5 years	Total	5-yr survival %
I	N−	24	25	97
	N+	35	37	
II	N−	26	26	72
	N+	51	72	
III	N−	16	21	29
	N+	16	52	
Total		158	233	68

Table 16. *Quantitative distribution of axillary metastases*

Grade	No. of N+ cases	Mean no. of nodes	Mean no. of nodes N+	No. of cases with only 1 node N+	No. of cases with massive involvment (more than 9 nodes N+)	No. of cases with capsular rupture
I	37	13	2.8	13	0	11
II	72	14	4	17	7	23
III	52	14	6	7	11	20

A study of 233 cases of adenocarcinoma of the breast initially operated, without prior irradiation, at the Institut Gustave-Roussy during the period 1954—1959 showed that there is a correlation between the grading and the 5-year survival rate, also a relationship between the quality and quantity of lymph node invasion.

Tables 14—17 show the various links discovered, according to the technique used to allocate the tumors to one category or the other.

Table 17. *Five-yr survival by T class and no. of N+ lymph nodes*

	No. of N+ lymph nodes			No. of
	1—3	4—6	More than 6	N+ cases
T1	23/26 (92%)	9/9 (100%)	2/2 (100%)	37
T2	39/48 (31%)	8/13 (62%)	4/12 (33%)	72
T3	8/23 (35%)	2/9 (22%)	5/18 (28%)	52

Thus, if specimens obtained from lymph-node dissection are available, it is possible to define three large groups with a decreasing probability of survival:

1. all cases in Grade I, whether N+ or N−; N− cases in Grade II, almost all of whom are alive after 5 years;

2. all N+ cases in Grade II; N− cases in Grade III, only 72% of whom are alive after 5 years;

3. N+ cases in Grade III, of whom a mere 29% survive after 5 years.

Furthermore, the number of lymph nodes invaded varies in parallel with the histological grade: an average of 2.8 in Grade I, as against 6 in Grade III. Conversely, there are very few cases in Grades II and III with a single lymph-node metastasis (17 out of 72 and 5 out of 52 respectively, a non-significant difference) and relatively more in Grade I (13 out of 37). Similarly, multiple metastases and cases with capsular rupture are much more numerous with tumors in Grade III.

A study of the survival rates for these various groups, although some of them do not contain enough cases to give a valid percentage (these are quoted in brackets), show that the prospects for Grade III tumors are poor, whatever the number of axillary lymph nodes involved.

It should be noted, however, that this grading does not allow for the qualitative or quantitative aspect of the stroma, certain aspects of which are able to modify this grading. Thus, of the 11 cases of "medullary carcinoma", or carcinoma limited to the lymphoid stroma, which form part of our series of 233 cases, eight come under Grade III, there being two in Grade II and none in Grade I; however, only one of them died within 5 years. This special stroma reaction may be a sign of host-tumor relationship, and thus may give a relatively more favorable prognosis in tumors of this type.

Conversely, we found that the size of the plaques of fibrinoid substance in the stroma of a carcinoma varied inversely with its histological grade; this type of stroma is frequent in Grade I, but seldom occurs in Grade III. However, statistical confirmation is needed and is being sought.

3. Biochemistry

The statistical study of breast cancer patients hospitalized at the Institut Gustave-Roussy between 1955 and 1959 enabled us to distinguish the following prognostic factors [15, 30].

1. With metastatic cancers, and cancers which are localized but with chest wall fixation, the patient's survival time is shorter the stronger the inflammatory reaction of the plasma. This inflammatory reaction of the plasma was studied at the Institut Gustave-Roussy mainly on the basis of the Resorcinol Index.

Balance sheets made out during each of these phases enable us to predict to some extent the course of events during subsequent stages and to modify treatment accordingly. Some of these predictions are more important than others. By and large, what interests the clinician most is the prediction of survival, so that this has been the subject of the majority of studies. We have, as already stated, directed our effort towards the investigation of criteria of prediction which can be of immediate help in the choice of therapy.

And finally, there will be some utility in predicting which patients with metastatic breast cancer are likely to benefit from hormone surgery, which is often disabling and should be strictly reserved for patients in whom it is likely to be effective. Nevertheless, it should be noted that the study of prognostic factors alone cannot determine which is the best treatment, and controlled therapeutic trials should be carried out to enable the various treatments to be compared.

2. Statistically, the survival time of breast cancer patients tends to be longer, the higher their blood cholesterol. This is a statistically significant concept for metastatic cancers. It is also found with localized forms, whether susceptible to surgery or not, but here the differences in the percentage of survivors are not significant in the various series studied. This antagonism appears to be due, not to the actual cholesterol, but to one or two biochemical factors which interfere with its endosynthesis. The confirmation of this phenomenon would appear to open up a new field of research. Moreover, in view of the enormous resources at present being devoted to the study of cholesterol synthesis and ways of modifying it, in an effort to mitigate the complications of atherosclerosis, there could well be some advantage in relating this research to the carcinological antagonism we have just mentioned.

4. Mastography

Out of a continuous series of 1009 patients with malignant breast cancer referred to the Institut Gustave-Roussy between 1st January, 1954, and 31st December, 1959, and treated at this center throughout, 432 had a radiological examination of the mammary gland [13, 27]. This examination, which was at first done only on selected patients, became routine from 1957 onwards, and we have confirmed that the group having radiography was representative of the patients treated at the Institut over the same period, more particularly that the extension of their cancer did not differ from that in subjects who were not radiographed.

We soon came to appreciate that, in addition to its diagnostic value, mastography undoubtedly has a prognostic value, too. This is the aspect to be discussed, looking first at the prognostic value of the various radiological features and then correlating them with the clinical features associated with survival.

a) Prognostic Value of Radiological Features

A study of the 1, 2, 3 and 4-year survival rates [13] showed that the following four features always indicate an unfavorable prognosis:

1. thickening of the nipple
2. thickening of the whole skin
3. edematous infiltration of the subcutis
4. edema of the gland.

Analyzing the results in still greater detail, we found that these features fall into two groups:

a) criteria 2. to 4. are very closely linked; if one is present, the other two usually are as well, and there is not much point in studying them separately. We have thus grouped them under the general term "malignant edema". The prognosis for patients presenting with these features is very unfavorable.

b) thickening of the nipple, on the other hand, can occur apart from any of the features of malignant edema; we observed 47 cases where this was so. But when it occurs alone, it seems to have no prognostic value. Its inclusion in the above criteria arises simply from the fact that thickening of the nipple is often associated with the "edematous" cluster. When this happens, survival rates are low, but the main cause of this is the edema.

This being the case, we shall discuss only the "malignant edematous" appearance, correlating it with the other prognostic criteria.

b) The "Malignant Edematous" Appearance

This radiological appearance (see Figs. 4—8) comprises three anomalies in association:

1. thickening of the skin;
2. infiltration and densification of the connective tissue-glandular region, designated by the term, edema of the gland;
3. an edematous infiltration of the subcutis, which loses its normal transparence and appears to be partitioned by thick trabeculi which form multiple small enclosures. At the same time the normal clear and regular boundaries between the subcutis, the skin and the connective tissue-glandular triangle become blurred.

This appearance is sometimes diffused and sometimes localized. It can be seen from a comparative radiological examination of both breasts. At first glance the affected breast gives an impression of densification. It must always be interpreted in the same way, whether or not it is associated with other radiological signs of malignity, such as tumoral opacities or microcalcifications. However, before accepting that this is the "malignant edematous" appearance, we must exclude cutaneous infiltrations of another kind, as observed in certain inflammatory conditions and after operation on the axilla or the mammary gland. In some cases discrete cutaneous and subcutaneous infiltrations occur which are pre-tumoral and difficult to distinguish from the "malignant edematous" appearance. However, we do after all distinguish them because the skin is less thickened, and the subcutis is not infiltrated but only the site of the strands of tissue connecting the tumor to the skin, which is sometimes retracted. Both these appearances are grouped under the heading, thickening of skin around the tumor, and we have found that they have no prognostic value.

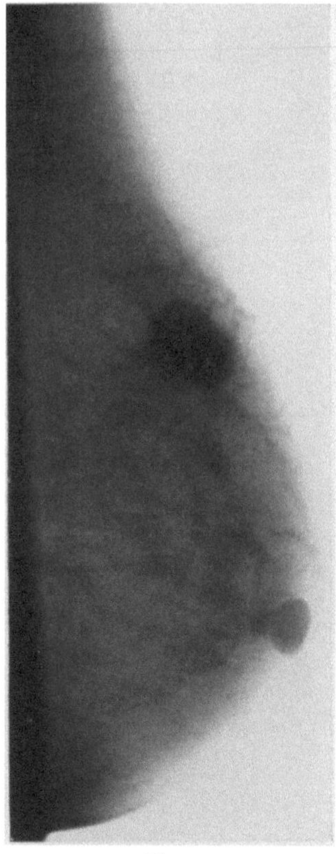
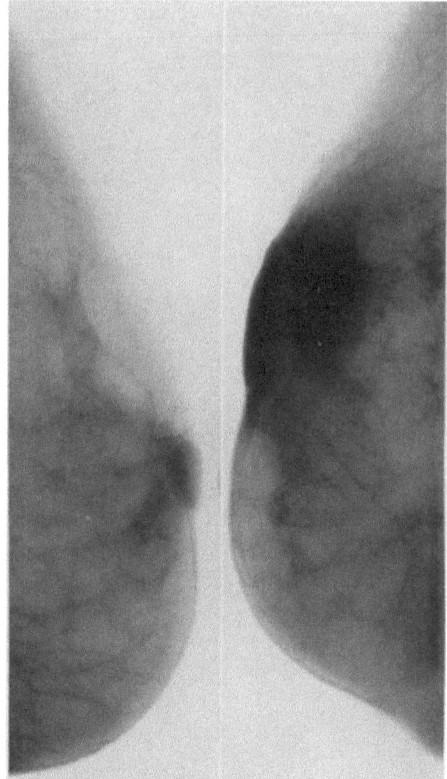

Fig. 4   Fig. 5

Fig. 4. *Case 05/59.4466, age 66 years.* Tumoral opacity of 2.5 cm over 2 cm of upper quadrant and median quadrant of left breast, roughly polylobular with regular contours. However, discrete infiltration of the subcutis and dilatation of the blood vessels round the tumor suggest malignity with localized edema. Operated and treated with [60]Co. In good health in Oct. 1968 at age 76

Fig. 5. *Case 05/61.5375, age 61 years.* Irregular tumoral opacity 3 cm in diameter in the subareolar region of the right breast. Limited skin thickening in the region of the nipple and localized subareolar edema can be seen. Operated in 1961 and treated with [60]Co. Many slowly developing bone metastases. Last seen Oct. 1968. General condition fairly good but in considerable pain

The "malignant edematous" appearance indicates an unfavorable prognosis equally for forms T1, T2, T3 and T4. In fact, if we group all cases, regardless of the T score, according to the picture of "malignant edema" and whether it is "localized" or total, we find the following 3-year survival rates:

344 cases without edema	82%
38 cases with the localized malignant edema picture	55%
45 cases with the total edema picture	9%

On the other hand, when the "malignant edematous" picture is present, the T score does not much affect the prognosis (Table 18).

Table 18. *Percentage with "malignant edematous aspect" according to T class*

	No. of cases	% with "malignant edema"
T1, T2	181	7
T3, T4	198	33

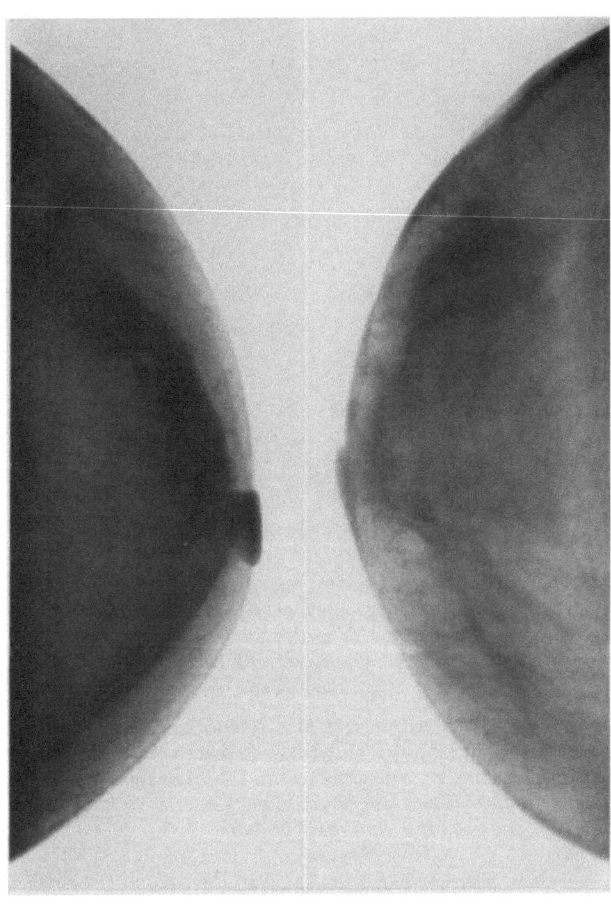

Fig. 6. *Case 05/61.4438, age 59 years.* Irregular opacity 3 cm in diameter in the supero-external quadrant of the right breast, containing a group of microcalcifications with edema of the subcutis and fairly general skin thickening, although worse in the outer quadrant. Sandwich course of ^{60}Co and operation—rapid development. Died within one year

5. Invasion of the Nipple

This study is based on 585 surgical specimens from which a systematic sampling was made in the region of the nipple, 3 or 4 sections being cut [28]. Twelve of these

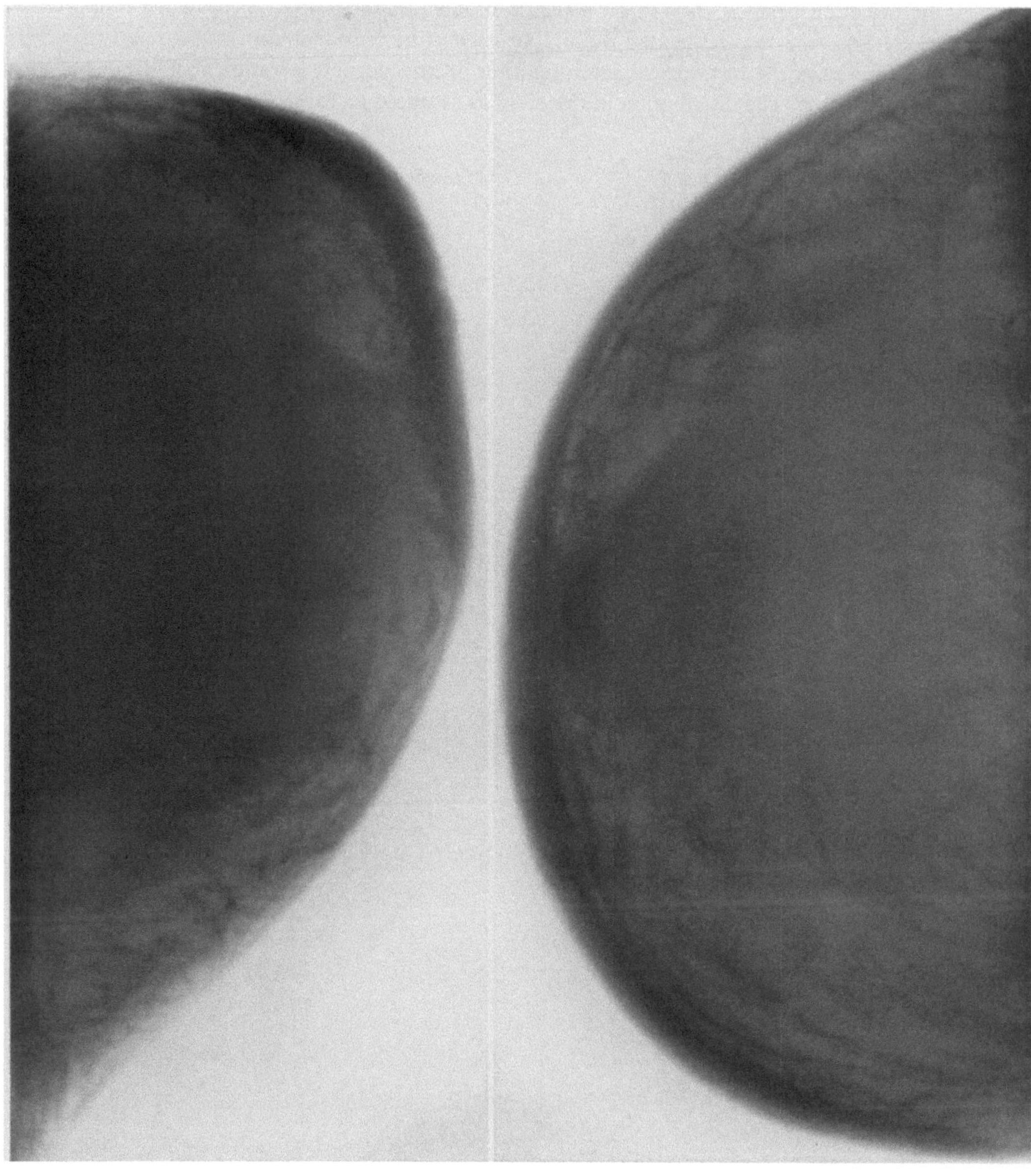

Fig. 7. *Case 05/62.1886, age 66 years.* Massive appearance of whole of left breast, with diffused edematous aspect and overall skin thickening. Treated with telecobalt (7000 rads) and mastectomy. Died after 4 years of continuing development

cases could not be correctly interpreted because of faulty fixing in this region. Furthermore, we should note that 37 cases belonged to an older series where low doses of radiation had been given before the operation; however, we think that when the radiation beam is focused on a tumor situated at some distance from the nipple (there are very few lesions of the nipple itself), the lesions it suffers are relatively mild and thus the histological interpretation of any possible invasion should not be too misleading. The distribution in this series is as stated in Table 19.

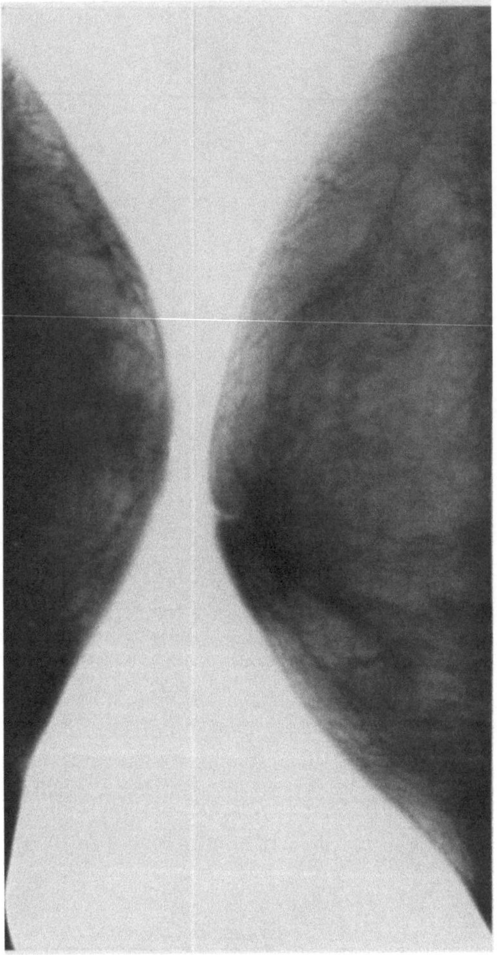

Fig. 8. *Case 05/60.6307, age 61 years.* Edematous aspect of both breasts, the left one being worse. Note invagination of both nipples

This table requires comment: it seems to be important that the clinician should differentiate between tumors which are wholly or partially located in the central or retro-mamillary region, which he can locate by palpation or by mammography, and "peripheral" tumors some way from the nipple, whose propagation in the nipple is discovered only at the time of the histological examination.

Table 19. *Breast cancer and invasion of or propagation to the nipple*

Invasion of nipple	No. of cases	5-yr survival %
Not known	12	
None	275	48
Histological only	195	34
Histological and clinical	103	18
Total	585	

Indeed, mamillary invasion by central or directly retro-mamillary tumors, or by massive tumors occupying the whole of the breast (42 cases in our series), can be considered as a neighborhood invasion, in the same way as one finds in proximity numerous tumoral nodules, duct propagations or small satellite neoplastic islets in the connective tissue, or embolisms in the lymphatics. The same occurs with mammary tumors situated in one quadrant but invading the central or retro-mamillary region (61 cases in our series). Such tumors come next in severity after central breast tumors; indeed, their severity may be even greater on account of the lymphatic drainage in this region.

The propagation in the nipple of tumors sited at a distance is quite a different matter (195 cases). It should be compared with the lesions of Paget's disease of the nipple, which almost always indicates a deep infiltrating tumor.

Four types of invasion or propagation in the nipple can be seen: the milk ducts, the lymphatics, invasion of the connective tissue, and intradermal propagation in the form of "Paget's" cells within the epidermis of the nipple. The following table shows how these various types are distributed in the case of "peripheral" tumors.

Table 20. *Routes of propagation to the nipple of tumors distant from it (467 cases)*

Propagation route	No. of cases Total	Only route	%
Ducts	137	106	23
Lymphatics	52	17	4
Interstitial	46	8	2
Paget or Paget-like	9	3	1
Multiple		49	10
None		284	60

Propagation via the milk ducts alone is by far the most frequent route for tumors distant from the central or retro-mamillary region (23%), propagation by multiple routes being considerably less frequent (10%), with the lymphatic, interstitial and epidermal routes a long way behind (4, 2 and 1% respectively).

We wished to see whether there was any connection between nipple propagations and the existence of axillary or retrosternal metastases. The next table shows the situation in our series (Table 21).

This table excludes 15 cases where the histological interpretation was doubtful, or where no lymph nodes had been taken out. Breaking these data down according to axillary or retrosternal involvement, we have the situation shown in Table 22.

Table 21. *Propagation to the nipple and lymph-node metastases*

Ax.	Int. Mam.	No propagation	Histological propagation	Histological + clinical	Total
N−	Not examined	19	8	2	29
N+	Not examined	21	15	7	43
N−	N−	67	28	17	112
N−	N+	9	5	1	15
N+	N−	113	76	45	234
N+	N+	44	63	30	137
Total		273	195	102	570

In cases of axillary invasion (Table 22), there is no significant difference when the propagation in the nipple is exclusively histological or when it is both clinical and histological.

Table 22. *Axillary invasion and propagation to the nipple*

	Invasion of axillary lymph nodes		
Propagation to the nipple	N+	N−	Total
None	178	95	273
Histological only	154	41	195
Histological + clinical	82	20	102
	414	156	570

p=0.01 **   NS=not significant

In cases of retrosternal invasion (Table 23), there is no significant difference when the tumor is under the nipple or in the central region and reaches the nipple by propagation. But for tumors distant from the nipple, propagation in the nipple is linked with retrosternal invasion (highly significant difference).

As shown by Table 24, there is no significant difference if we consider all tumors of inner quadrants in relation to outer tumors. However, if we consider just the supero-internal and supero-external quadrants, we find a significant difference in propagation within the nipple: 46% of supero-external as against 32% of supero-internal tumors.

Among these patients only one third were treated long enough ago to allow a correct evaluation of survival rates in the various categories. We have therefore attempted to assess the type of mamillary invasion, not in relation to survival but in relation to the axillary involvement whose excellent prognostic value is well known.

In cases of invasion by the milk ducts alone, the number of axillary lymph nodes invaded is more or less the same as where there is no invasion of the nipple; in cases of interstitital or lymphatic invasion, there are many more invaded lymph nodes.

Table 23. *Retrosternal invasion and propagation to the nipple*

Propagation to the nipple	Invasion of internal mammary chain		
	N+	N−	Total
None	53	180	233
Histological only	68	104	172
Histological+clinical	31	62	93
Total	152	346	498

Table 24. *Propagation to the nipple by distant tumors*

Tumor site	Propagation to the nipple		
	None	Hist. only	Total
Inner half	91	52	143
External half	128	96	224 NS
	219	148	367

Moreover, interstitial or lymphatic invasion is found more frequently where the volume of the tumor is greater, its fixation stronger and a greater number of lymph nodes are involved. All these features have a distinct prognostic value, so that we have asked ourselves whether, under these conditions, interstitial or lymphatic invasion of the nipple could constitute a supplementary factor in the prognosis. To answer this question, we have compared tumors of similar volume, some of which had interstitial or lymphatic nipple invasion, while the others had not. Those with nipple invasion were found to have lower survival rates than those without.

Proceeding in the same manner for tumor fixation and axillary invasion, we reached the conclusion that lymphatic or interstitial invasion of the nipple has a lower survival rate, irrespective of the clinical extension of the tumor or the condition of the axillary lymph nodes. It therefore has a prognostic value in its own right, independently of the other criteria. (Note, however, that these results were obtained from a small number of cases and are often at the limit of statistical significance, and they still have to be confirmed.)

Continuing our comparisons, we considered whether clinical extension or axillary invasion retain their prognostic value when the nipple is invaded (by the lymphatic or interstitial route) or not. It would appear that they do.

This whole set of comparisons regrouped within the framework of the TNM system enabled us to construct Table 25, which confirms the prognostic value of the pathological state of the nipple. Summing up, therefore, we would say that, although

Table 25. *Five-yr survival rate related to invasion of nipple for different extensions according to T*

T	No propagation or by ducts only		Lymphatic or interstitial propagation		Significance after weighting
	No. of cases	5-yr surv.	No. of cases	5-yr surv.	
T1, T2	67	78%	16	63%	*
T3, T4	8	63%	13	23%	

p=0.05 *

invasion of the nipple plays an important part in the prognostic process independently of the familiar criteria, these still retain a very definite value.

6. Number of Lymph Nodes Invaded

Axillary chain. Clearly, we have verified that patients whose axillary lymph nodes are invaded have a more serious form of the disease than the others. In addition, we have found that the more lymph nodes invaded, the lower the survival rate (Table 26). This is especially clear in the 5-year survival study: women having only one affected node have survival rates very close to those of patients with no axillary metastases, while after this there is a fairly regular decline [35].

Table 26. *Survival rate related to axillary invasion*

Survival (years)	1		2		3		4		5	
	cases	%	cases	%	cases	%	cases	%	cases	%
No. of lymph nodes invaded										
0	108	99	94	95	80	91	62	89	39	92
1	60	97	45	91	36	89	26	88	14	86
2	45	96	37	86	32	81	24	71	13	69
3	32	100	30	97	25	88	17	71	12	58
4—5	27	93	24	83	18	72	13	77	10	70
6—7	31	100	29	86	23	78	19	68	10	60
$\geq$ 8	33	91	29	66	25	56	18	50	13	31
Significance of the regression			**		***		***		***	

p=0.05 *   p=0.01 **   p $\leq$ 0.001 ***

This result was verified on cases where only one lymph node was invaded by excluding that one lymph node.

It seemed worth considering minor invasions (one lymph node): these include a fairly large number of "hidden" metastases consisting in neoplastic embolisms at the level of the sinus, or the presence of a few cancer cells in other parts of the lymph node. The prognosis in such cases is as favorable as for non-invasive forms.

Taking all these results together, we are led to suppose that the extent of axillary involvement plays an important part in establishing the prognosis.

Internal mammary chain. As with the axillary chain, there is a very clear link between survival and the number of lymph nodes invaded (Table 27).

Table 27. *Survival rate related to invasion of the internal mammary chain*

Survival (years)	1		2		3	
	cases	%	cases	%	cases	%
No. of lymph nodes invaded						
0	86	99	64	95	48	90
1—2	36	97	32	81	28	71
3	14	86	13	62	9	56
Significance of the regression	*		***		**	

p=0.05 *   p=0.01 ** $p \leq 0.001$ ***

7. Clinical Dimensions and Radiological Dimensions

Clinicians are concerned with the problem of assessing the true size of the tumor, particularly in view of the importance of this criterion in the TNM classification. The volume of the breast and the thickness of the skin introduce variables, and there are others. So we have considered whether measuring the radiological picture would enable us to come to grips with this problem. We therefore compared the radiological size with the clinical size and studied the results to see whether the difference had any prognostic value. The measurements were carried out on 303 cases, subdivided into three groups according to the diameter of the tumor.

a) in the 38 cases where clinical and radiological dimensions were the *same*, the 5-year survival rate is 79%.

On breaking these cases down by size, we found:

1—2 cm   (8 cases) 5-yr survival rate 100%
3—5 cm (23 cases) 5-yr survival rate 83%
over 5 cm   (7 cases) 5-yr survival rate 43%

Thus, size alone has a strong prognostic value.

b) In cases where the clinical size was *bigger* than the radiological one, we found that the difference between the two supplied additional information which is by no means negligible. Our findings were:

over 1 cm (98 cases) 5-yr survival rate 82%
over 2 cm (86 cases) 5-yr survival rate 69%
over 3 cm (47 cases) 5-yr survival rate 57%
over 4 cm (30 cases) 5-yr survival rate 60%

F. Extent of Surgical Intervention

This factor varies as a function of the initial clinical form of the disease, whether pre-operative radiation was done or not, and the condition of the lymph nodes. In addition to the initial biopsy on which the histological diagnosis is based, four types of operation are carried out at the Institut Gustave-Roussy:

1. simple mastectomy;
2. mastectomy with axillary dissection and conservation of the pectoral muscles (Patey's technique);
3. the classic Halsted technique;
4. Halsted's operation with internal mammary dissection.

1. Simple Mastectomy

This operation consists in the ablation of the tumor and the entire mammary gland. We use an oval incision with a broad horizontal axis circumscribing the breast. This transverse incision is easier to suture, especially in thin women, as the skin flaps can be more easily stretched. As regards comfort and esthetics, the mobility of the shoulder is easier to preserve and the scar will in no way interfere with it. The conservation of the muscle mass and the low level of the incision have undeniable esthetic advantages for the patient. Early and rapid cicatrization (necrosis of the flaps hardly ever occurs) means that post-operative irradiation can be given without delay, should it prove necessary.

The skin flaps are loosened at top and bottom to the outer limits of the gland, which is excised down to the level of the aponeurosis of the pectoralis major. This operation also allows a low sample to be taken from the axillary nodes so that a histological check can be made on the external mammary lymph nodes.

If the tumor is fixed to the pectoralis major or its aponeurosis (T3 and T4 tumors), the muscular zones involved are excised as well, especially when simple mastectomy is being carried out to remove tumoral vestiges remaining after radiotherapy.

2. Mastectomy with Axillary Dissection (Patey's Technique)

Two types of incision may be used:

a) the transverse incision, as used for simple mastectomy. It is merely extended further to the rear, or inclined slightly upwards towards the external part of the axilla, and then, after the skin flaps have been loosened over a wide area, it is quite easy to get at the axilla.

b) an oblique incision, circumscribing the tumor and ending at the top on the anterior face of the pectoralis major, a little way inside its external margin. The axillary dissection is done first and, if it is desired to have it as complete as possible, we recommend cutting the tendon of the pectoralis minor to give readier access to the top of the axillary pyramid. Nevertheless, dissection under these conditions is a little more difficult than with Halsted's operation. The supero-internal portion of the axillary fat should be marked with a clip or colored thread, also the supero-internal limit of the mass of cells and lymph nodes. This procedure enables the axillary fat to be orientated in the required direction and allows a topographical study to be made of the step-by-step lymph node invasion (see p. 12).

3. Radical Amputation of the Breast or Halsted's Technique

Our technique differs very little from that described by HALSTED in 1889, and then only in the types of incision used and the closing of the skin flaps.

We use an almost vertical incision, starting at the top of the subclavicular cutaneous depression at the level of the coracoid process, circumscribing the tumor and finishing at the inferior margin of the thorax. This incision usually makes for easy closing, as the skin flaps are loosened over a wide area; above all, as it does not encroach on the axilla, it may avoid the creation of any retractile ligament which could interfere with abduction of the arm.

There is, of course, no standard incision and the cut can be modified according to the site of the tumor, particularly since we always resect 5 cm of skin on either side of the tumor.

The skin flaps are loosened internally as far as the sternum and externally as far as the external face of the dorsalis major, at the top as far as the clavicle, and at the bottom as far as the aponeurosis of the rectus abdomini. The tendon of the pectoralis major is cut on the outside level with its brachial insertion, as an unduly economical cut will leave an ugly bulge behind at the level of the muscle stumps. Once the aponeurosis is open, the pectoralis minor is also cut at the level of its coracoid insertion. The dissection of the axillary packet is simple once the muscular covering of the armpit has been laid open, and the mass of cells and lymph nodes can be removed without difficulty.

We nearly always leave intact the nerves of the latissimus dorsi and deltoid muscles.

After a very careful hemostasis, the skin is closed, generally without excessive traction. The insertion of a drain under depression, enabling the skin tension to be relaxed, has greatly reduced the number of post-operative hematomas and lymphorrhagias, as well as necrosis of the flaps.

4. Extended Operation: Halsted + Internal Mammary Dissection

Our Institut was the first, under our master, H. REDON, to introduce this operation into France 20 years ago. Even at that time there had been some more extensive operations, combining radical ablation of the mammary gland and pectoral muscles with triple curettage—axillary, mammary and supraclavicular. We gave up triple curettage, as the follow-up of a series of 20 patients showed that, in the case of supraclavicular invasion, survival time was less than 2 years. Thus, invasion of the supraclavicular lymph nodes, a second relay stage invasion, had an unfavorable prognosis and was considered beyond help by surgical exeresis.

We thus restricted the surgical procedure to double dissection, axillary and internal mammary, removing nodes which had been directly invaded by the medium of the main axillary lymphatic and accessory internal mammary lymphatic routes.

Internal mammary dissection is done first, after the loosening of the internal cutaneous flap. It comprises ablation of the 2nd, 3rd and 4th costal cartilages and exeresis of the mass of cells and lymph nodes in the first four intercostal spaces, together with the internal mammary vessels. It is an extra-pleural dissection, passing under the endothoracic fascia but sparing the pleura behind it. The depression resulting from this dissection, which is unesthetic, troublesome and very liable to unfortunate sequelae, is filled in by muscular flaps taken from the clavicular head of the pectoralis major by severing its external attachments and turning it downwards and inwards by rotating it around its internal sterno-clavicular attachments.

The procedure is completed by Halsted's technique, including the axillary dissection.

It is still too soon to be able to judge the therapeutic value of these extended operations, but an international therapeutic trial is currently being undertaken at the Institut Gustave-Roussy and several other national centers. This will enable long-term results to be compared for two sets of patients, allocated at random, one treated by Halsted's operation and the other by Halsted's operation combined with internal mammary dissection.

G. The Techniques of Radiotherapy

Local/regional irradiation comprises continuous irradiation of the primary tumor, its local/regional propagation (chest wall and mammary gland, if necessary) and its lymphatic diffusion [42, 60].

The subcutaneous and glandular lymphatics of the breast fall under three relay routes (see Fig. 9):

1. *axillary,* comprising four main groups (A, B, C, D);

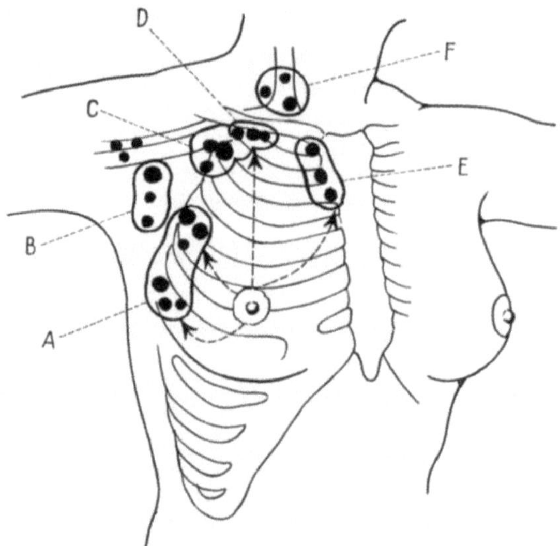

Fig. 9. *Location of mammary lymphatics*

First relay level:	axillary	
	A	external mammary
	B	scapular
	C	central or intermediate
	D	retro-clavicular or apical
Second relay level:	E	internal mammary
Third relay level:	F	supra-clavicular

2. *internal* mammary (E), here the maximum risk of invasion is at the level of the first three intercostal spaces;

3. *supraclavicular* (F), this level is reached by either the internal or external route, by way of the other relay stages.

The conception of local/regional irradiation differs according to the indications, of which there are five:

as part of the initial treatment — combined with surgery — 1. pre- and 2. post-operatively; 3. local, when the cancer is limited to the breast or 4. functional, when there are distant metastases; or 5. when it is utilized for parietal or lymphatic recurrence.

1. Post-operative Radiotherapy

This technique is typical of local/regional irradiation.

Telecobalt has been in current use for some ten years and has been applied in all cases of mammary irradiation at the Institut Gustave-Roussy since 1960. If the first few millimeters of tissue to be traversed are given a sub-dose, this prevents both immediate and subsequent cutaneous reactions, such as frequently occur when large surfaces are to be irradiated. Its yield in depth facilitates the irradiation of lymph node volumes and reduces the dose to the superficial layers while delivering an equivalent dose to the tumor.

Four *target volumes* are included in post-operative irradiation, representing the local/regional dissemination of the mammary carcinoma (Figs. 10, 11, 12):

volume B = scar and chest wall

C = homologous axillary lymph nodes

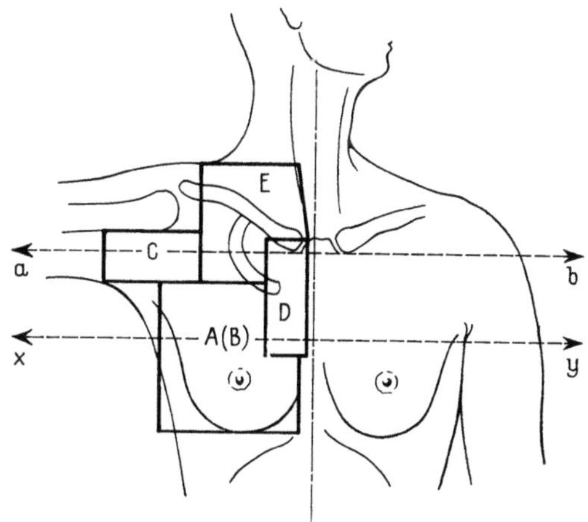

Fig. 10. *Target volumes seen in frontal view of the patient*

A   primary tumor and breast
B   subjacent thoracic wall
C   axilla
D   homolateral internal mammary chain
E   supra-clavicular

Transverse sections through *xy* (Fig. 11) and *ab* (Fig. 12) show the configuration in depth of the volumes in the tissues

E = supraclavicular lymphatic plexus
D = homolateral internal mammary chain

These volumes are irradiated by means of five *fields:* two of these are the internal (Fig. 11) and external (Fig. 12) tangential thoracic fields, the other three being designed to reach the lymph nodes (anterior supraclavicular, anterior axillary and posterior axillary — Figs. 13 and 14).

Careful irradiation of the axilla and the retroclavicular region should always be carried out; because the nodes extend so deeply, one third or one quarter of the axillary volume must be administered from a posterior field (Fig. 15).

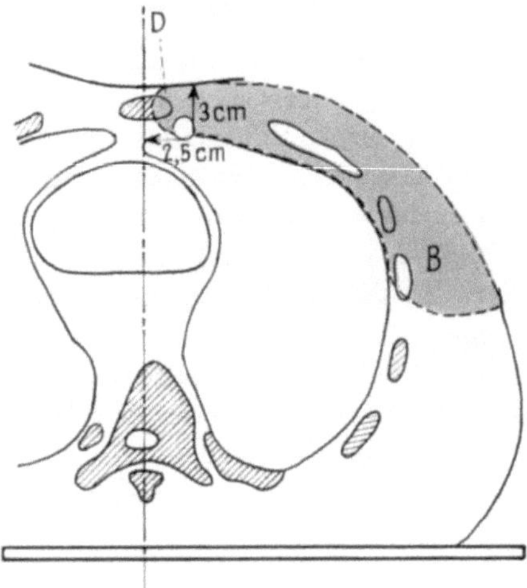

Fig. 11. *Target volumes along a transverse section at the level of the chest wall (xy in Fig. 10)*

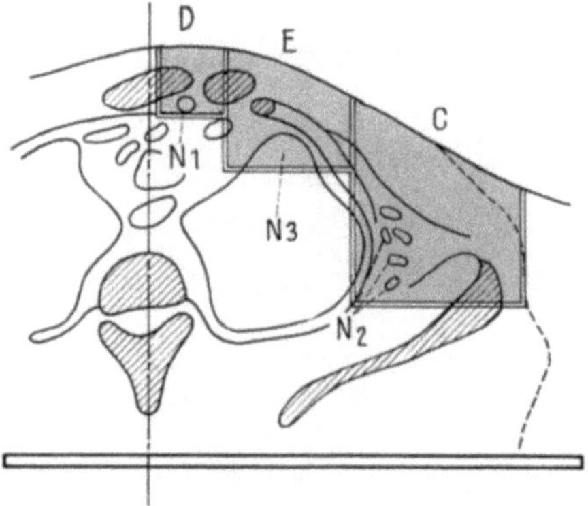

Fig. 12. *Target volumes along a transverse section at the level of the internal mammary lymph nodes (ab in Fig. 10). Close to the median line can be seen volume D (internal mammary chain), on the outside volume C (axillary lymph nodes) and between the two, volume E (supra- and retro-clavicular region)*

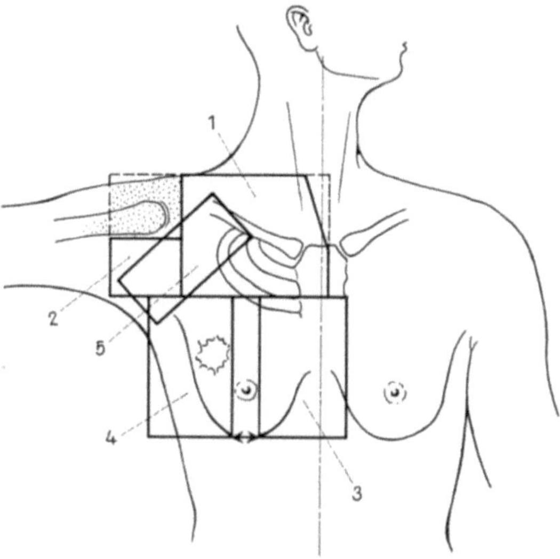

Fig. 13. *Telecobalt therapy: fields used for local/regional irradiation of breast carcinoma*

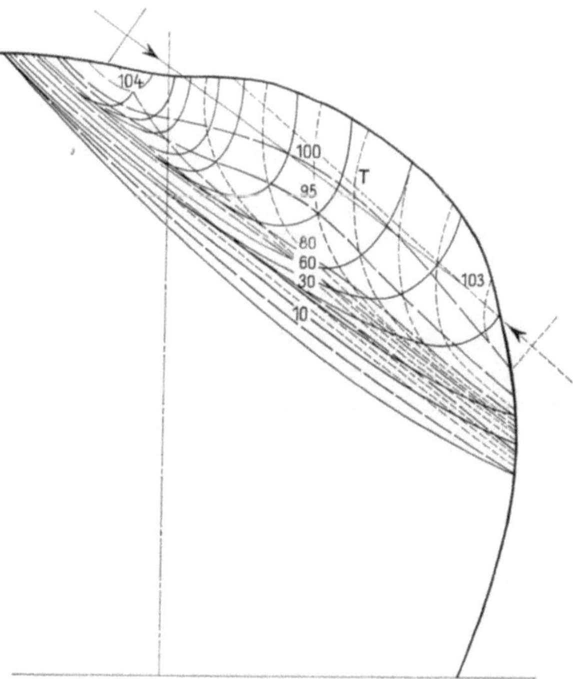

Fig. 14. *Isodose curves of the thoracic wall.* These are irradiated by an internal tangential field (305°) and an external tangential field (130°) in order to spare the lung as much as possible

It is equally important not to underdose the parasternal region, either because the operation was for simple mastectomy or because the invaded lymph nodes have been removed by internal mammary dissection.

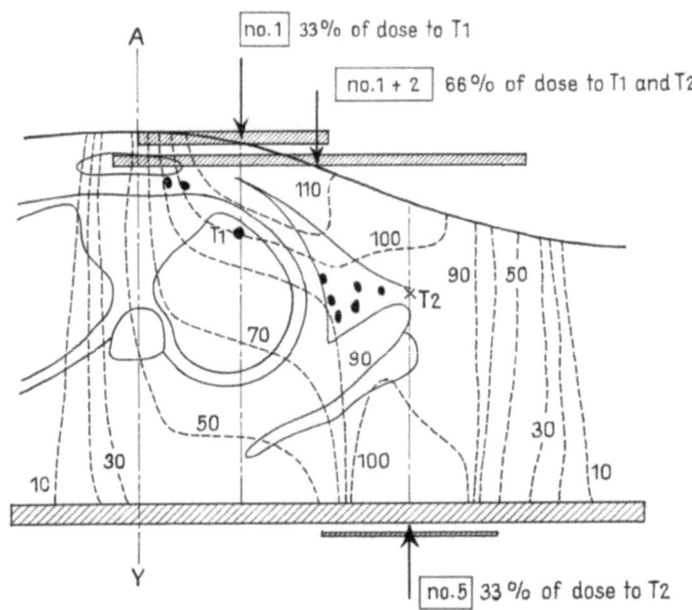

Fig. 15. *Distribution of the dose within the tissues* (transverse section through plane *ab* of Fig. 10). The large field (Nos. 1 and 2) covers both the supra-clavicular and axillary regions and delivers 66% of the dose to points T1 and T2. Field No. 1 is directed at the clavicular region and the first homologous internal mammary space and delivers 33% of the dose to point T1. Field No. 5, posterior axillary, completes the treatment of the axillary region and delivers 33% of the dose to point T2

Irradiation of the contralateral internal mammary chain, although recommended by some authors, is not done at the Institut Gustave-Roussy because it involves a substantial degree of irradiation of the lungs and the normal breast.

A dose of 4500 rads is given over a period of one month to the whole of the target volumes.

2. Pre-operative Radiotherapy

The target volumes comprise, over and above those irradiated post-operatively, the breast and the primary tumor. The beams used are the same. The tissue dose is 4500 rads over one month for all volumes where treatment is to be supplemented by surgical resection (breast and axilla), or for those where the risk of invasion is slight (supraclavicular depression). The internal mammary chain has a strong likelihood of being pathological with internal or central tumors so, where it is not to be dissected, it should be superdosed to the level of the first three intercostal spaces, which should receive 6000 rads.

3. Regional Radiotherapy alone

Treatment is carried out in two stages:

a) initial irradiation by the pre-operative technique, which is the same for all patients, taken to 4500 rads in all volumes;

b) complementary irradiation adapted to each individual case and effected by means of fields superimposed on the broad beams given earlier. These superimposed fields, which are kept as low as possible, are given for palpable remnants of the primary tumor and in the armpit (Fig. 16). The first three mammary spaces are always superdosed for central or internal tumors. Supraclavicular remnants are irradiated as required by small direct fields.

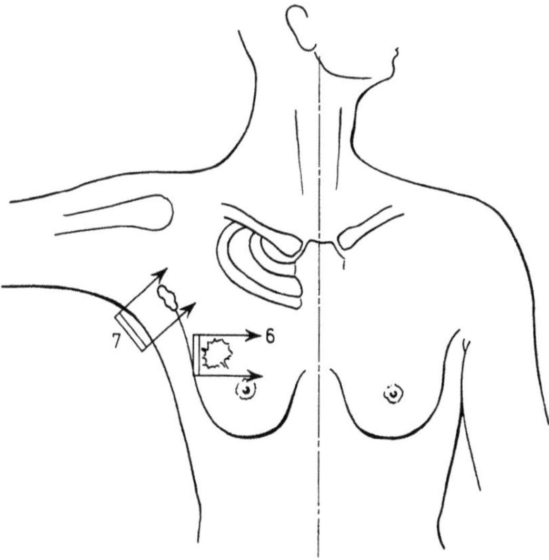

Fig. 16. *Superimposed direct axillary and external irradiation of the primary tumor, supplementing the doses already given where remnants of lesions are found*

Certain residual mammary tumors require a very heavy dose of radiation which is obtained only with difficulty by the external route; this is a good indication for interstitial curietherapy, which ought to be done if the condition of the lymph nodes offers a good hope of long survival.

The extra dose given varies for each patient, depending on her general condition, the extent of the residual lesions and the patient's tolerance of irradiation, from 2500 rads over 2 weeks to 3500 rads over 3 weeks. There seems to be an optimum dose which combines the maximum effect on the tumor with the least number of sequelae and which appears to fall within the range of 7000—8000 rads over 6—8 weeks and in 30—40 sessions.

4. Castration by Irradiation

The techniques reported in the literature are remarkable in their diversity and sometimes in their lack of precision, too. We shall not review them here, but only describe the technique used at the Institut Gustave-Roussy with which we have obtained consistent results. Three parameters come into play: the volume irradiated, the dose, and the duration of the irradiation.

The volume irradiated covers the whole of the pelvis. It extends 1 cm beyond the right and left bony margins where the pelvis is widest and it extends towards the feet as far as the pubic symphysis and towards the head as far as the promontory. This volume is irradiated by means of two fields: anterior pelvic and posterior pelvic, opposed. The fields measure 10—12 cm along the head/foot axis and 13—15 cm across it, according to the patient's physical build. The amount of radiation administered is calculated on the frontal plane of the pelvis. A study of the distribution of the dose within the tissues shows that, with the telecobalt which we use, this distribution is more or less homogeneous between the two portals. Distribution is not very different with adequately filtered conventional radiation (CDA: 2 mm Cu), at least in patients whose body thickness is less than 22 cm. For the others, the technique can be modified by the addition of two lateral fields to ensure that the ovaries receive the planned dose while the cutaneous reaction remains acceptable.

The dose and the spacing are interdependent. They vary according to whether castration is carried out at the same time as post-operative irradiation, or on its own. In the first case, we are dealing with patients already attending the radiotherapy department for local/regional irradiation. There is thus no difficulty in spacing the irradiation of the ovaries. 1500 rads are given over 2—3 weeks at a rate of 2 sessions per week.

In the second case, where castration alone is being done, the spacing is reduced to less than one week. Women who are near or have reached the menopause have 3 sessions and younger women 4. A dose of 300 rads is given at each session, so that the total dose received by the ovaries is from 900—1200 rads in 3 or 5 days.

Two points should be noted: first, it is wise to carry out a preliminary gynecological examination to make sure that there is no large mass within the pelvis which could modify the position of the ovaries; second, it is absolutely necessary to make radiographic checks with the same radiation beam which is to be used for the treatment, in order to ensure that the radiation field really covers the pelvis and hence the target volume as defined. Such a check is even more imperative with obese women whose skin is very mobile. Most of the failures of castration by irradiation are certainly due either to faulty ballistics or to an inadequate dose. To observe strict discipline at the technical level certainly provides insurance against such failures. The menopause can be achieved by a simple irradiation which is not distressing to the patient and, if a few elementary rules are observed, is always effective.

H. Hormone Therapy

1. Androgens

The use of male hormone is accompanied by grave disadvantages which must be emphasized, because one must take into consideration, not only the prospect of a brief improvement, but also the general well-being of the patient.

At therapeutic doses, which are of the order of 50—100 mg per day of testosterone propionate, the patient soon notices unpleasant side-effects. Nausea, vomiting and water retention are some of the least upsetting of these. What we consider more serious are above all the signs of virilization, which include gruffness of voice, growth of hair (hyperpilosity), redness of the face, acne and increased libido. It may be thought odd that we include these symptoms among the more serious complications although they do not endanger life. Our attitude will not, however, surprise anyone having a wide experience of consultations with breast cancer sufferers and who has won his patients' confidence to the extent that they talk freely. A woman afflicted with cancer of the breast has usually since her illness was detected been subjected to a series of physical and psychic stresses which have disturbed her profoundly. Mastectomy alone is a distressing experience, leaving her with the feeling that she is now less of a woman. She will have recovered her poise only with difficulty. Should the discovery of a metastasis undermine it again by requiring the use of a form of treatment likely to rob her of the last shreds of her femininity?

While it is possible to hide the scar of HALSTED's procedure so that a woman can be seen in public without her loss being suspected, her feminine pride is thrown into complete disarray by the results of taking androgens. Worse still, this is likely to induce an enhanced sexual drive which, particularly in the older woman, constantly aggravates the emotional difficulties and is radically opposed to the calm state of mind she needs to come to terms with her illness. Male hormones are cruel drugs, and they will have to show proof of a stronger therapeutic effect than has so far been observed before doctors will use them despite their masculinizing effects and the mental suffering which follows.

Furthermore, it appears that under some vaguely defined circumstances androgens may break down into estrogens within the organism, thus constituting an indirect form of estrogen treatment which may well aggravate the lesions in the younger woman.

For all these reasons, systematic androgen treatment has been completely discarded from the list of treatments for breast cancer used at the Institut Gustave-Roussy. There is, however, one exception and one reservation. On the one hand, under-nourished patients may be given "weakly masculinizing" androgens, such as the derivatives of 19-nortestosterone, for their anabolizing effects and in order to bring about a temporary restoration of general condition. On the other hand, several "para-androgens" have been introduced in recent years and it is claimed that they combine a substantial anti-cancer activity with negligible virilizing effects. Δ-1-Testolactone is said to be among these. However, it has not yet been available long enough to be evaluated. Should it indeed fulfil these claims, the above criticisms of androgens would, of course, become obsolete.

2. Estrogens

These hormones should be reserved exclusively for women well past the menopause. The risks of aggravating cancer in the younger woman by treating her with estrogens are no longer in doubt. It is, moreover, equally certain that the abuse of estrogens at the period of the menopause has been responsible, if not for the induction, at least for the stimulation of a previously quiescent breast cancer. In practical terms, we use estrogens only in women over 55 whose vaginal smears have been cytologically checked to make sure that all natural estrogen production has ceased.

No one particular estrogen seems to be better than another; primarily synthetic estrogens are used, either hexestrol or diethyl stilbestrol, in daily doses of the order of 25—50 mg, or ethinyl estradiol in doses of 1—3 mg. We should mention incidentally that, unlike other hormone treatments habitually used for mammary carcinoma, these doses have nothing in common with those which control the natural hormone balance of the organism, being of the order of 100—1000 times higher. This may well be one of the oblique aspects from which the mechanisms of action of hormone therapy ought to be compared with that of chemotherapy.

Lesions of the soft tissues are those which most often respond, then visceral lesions, and lastly bone metastases. Estrogen therapy brings with it a certain number of side-effects of a more or less distressing nature: pigmentation, nausea, vomiting, dysuria, metrorrhagia, which can occur during or after treatment. Accumulated sodium retention may aggravate an already precarious cardiovascular condition. True, this last complication is rare if the precaution is taken with any woman whose cardiovascular state is in doubt of prescribing along with these hormones a low-sodium diet and regular checks on her blood pressure.

In any case, these risks and discomforts are in no way comparable with those caused by male hormone. They are not sufficient to discredit estrogen therapy, which we consider a most useful weapon in our armamentarium.

Does para-oxypropiophenone deserve a special place among the estrogens? Apparently not. It was claimed to have a weak estrogenic action relative to its inhibitory action on the hypophysis. We consider, however, that this product should be classed with all other estrogens and hence its use should be banned in younger women with breast cancer.

3. Progesterone

Progesterone made a somewhat later appearance among the drugs used in breast cancer. Most authors attribute a 20—25% efficacy to it. We ourselves have recorded nine remissions among 38 patients treated. These remissions usually occur with lesions of the soft tissues; they are seldom prolonged. We know of one patient with peritoneal lesions who had 20 months' remission, but this appears to be exceptional. As a rule the benefits induced by progesterone are far less definite. Two facts must be stressed: (1) the extraordinary tolerance of the organism towards this hormone—at the usual therapeutic doses, which are of the order of 6 g per month with hydroxy-progesterone caproate, there are generally very few side-effects; (2) progesterone, or the synthetic progestogens such as lyndiol, has an enhanced therapeutic effect when combined with estrogens. This is a matter to which we shall return later.

4. The Steroids

Steroid therapy is one of the most valuable weapons at the carcinologist's disposal in his fight against locally extensive or metastatic mammary lesions.

Excluding replacement therapy following adrenalectomy or hypophysectomy, there are three therapeutic dose ranges for steroid therapy.

a) *High doses of steroids* (75—200 mg of cortisone hemisuccinate daily). These high doses are generally required to treat short-term emergency states, such as coma due to cerebral metastases or pulmonary or pleural metastases producing acute dyspnea.

b) *Moderate doses of steroids* (50 mg of cortisone or 25—30 mg of prednisone daily). The development of the tumor is not affected and we cannot expect regression under this type of treatment. But the anti-inflammatory effect of the hormone often brings about functional improvements which can be extremely beneficial. Bone metastases and pleuro-pulmonary metastases benefit most from this treatment. It is not rare to see severe ostalgias and dramatic dyspneas disappear within 24 hours of treatment.

The acute metastatic febrile syndromes are similarly influenced, often in the most spectacular manner. A metastatic febrile episode which has been fluctuating around 39—40° for weeks may disappear within a few hours. It bears repeating, however, that it would be wrong to consider steroid therapy as an anti-neoplastic treatment in the true sense of the words. But even with this reservation, steroid therapy under such circumstances remains one of the most effective forms of treatment available for restoring the patient's comfort.

Certain facts may appear to invalidate the above conclusions, i. e. that the functional benefit so obtained is accompanied at these doses by an antimitotic effect producing regression of the lesion. The behavior under steroid treatment of serous effusions in the pleura or peritoneum often tends to give this impression. One does, in fact, often observe ascites or pleurisy regressing or drying up under steroids; in cases of pulmonary metastases it is equally common to see a patent radiological improvement of parenchymal lesions. Similarly, the neurological disorders brought about by a cerebral metastasis often clear up after a perfusion of cortisone hemiscuccinate. But these facts need interpreting. We must not forget that some neoplastic foci become surrounded by inflammation and that this may be responsible for some of the patient's discomfort and for chest X-rays which show extensive lesions surrounding a cancerous core of much smaller size. Similarly, certain serous effusions are less the effect of the cancer itself than of the inflammatory reaction which surrounds it. In such cases, the steroid treatment appears to act by reducing this inflammatory area. Although we should be deceiving ourselves if we were to suppose that the malignant foci recede to the same extent, there is no doubt that the patient benefits, even if only for a time, and this must not be underestimated.

c) *Low-dose steroid therapy* (20 mg of cortisone or 10 mg of prednisone daily). These doses may be used either to continue over a longer period a steroid treatment which has proved its worth at higher doses, or to complement castration and inhibit the initiation of compensatory cortico-adrenal hyperproduction.

We have so far considered steroid therapy only in terms of cortisone and prednisone, these being the two products of which we have the most experience. It seems that there is no particular objection to using the related products: methyl prednisone, betamethasone, dextramethasone etc., in the corresponding anti-inflammatory doses.

In spite of the often spectacular efficacy of steroid therapy, some physicians hesitate to use it. Their reluctance stems from a double fear. First, they say, the hormone may carry a risk of increased osteolysis; second, it may reduce the patient's immunological defenses and hence her potential resistance to the disease of cancer. At the practical level, we consider both these fears to be unfounded. It is a well-known fact that cortisone can cause osteoporosis; this is one of the classic symptoms of Cushing's disease. Therefore it is logical *a priori* to fear that steroids will aggravate the skeletal changes caused by neoplastic involvement of the bones. In point of fact, this simply does not happen; we cannot recall a single patient in whom steroid therapy manifestly worsened the pre-existing bone lesions of mammary origin. It should indeed be remembered that osteoporosis of steroid origin is frequently the result of months and even years of hormone treatment. But above all it seems that in the matter of bone metastases due to breast cancer, a dual antagonistic process sets in. On the one hand we have the classic process of the liberation of calcium due to the direct impact of the hormone on the bone, and on the other an inhibition of the osteolytic action. This dual action generally ensures the neutralization of the bone-degrading process. When massive doses of cortisone are given, the latter process might even prevail over the former; this would explain the recalcification of osteolyses. Whatever the nature of this still poorly understood relationship, we can at least say that the fear of aggravating mammary osteolyses by steroid treatment appears to be unfounded.

The problem of the weakening of immunological defenses by steroids is doubtless even more complex. So far as we know, there has been no work done on this. The extinction of the B.C.G. reaction in patients receiving cortisone has been observed at the Institut Gustave-Roussy, but there is no evidence that the defenses against cancer are affected by it, at any rate where breast cancer is concerned. Furthermore, we have shown that this situation does not arise until daily doses of 40 mg or more of prednisone are given, and this is well above the routine therapeutic level. The risk certainly seems in this case to be more apparent than real.

Naturally, steroids should not be prescribed without good reason. The risks of internal hemorrhage, of inducing diabetes, or neuro-psychic disorders, and of fluid retention have to be taken into consideration. They call for stringent precautions and constant supervision; but they are not sufficient to discredit steroid therapy which we consider in general terms one of the most effective treatments for use in overcoming functional difficulties arising out of the metastases due to breast cancer.

5. Combined Therapy

We have recourse, in combination with steroid therapy, to the more manageable synthetic estrogens and progestogens, such as lyndiol, the combination of mestranol and lynestrol widely used in contraceptive pills. This combination is usually well tolerated; vaginal bleeding is the complication which arises most often. Signs of digestive intolerance may also occasionally be observed. But in general this treatment is well accepted.

These combinations do, however, raise certain questions. We mention here some which we think important.

1. Does the addition of a steroid to the estrogen/progestogen pair increase the therapeutic value of the method, as has been claimed? We know of no work done to determine whether this is actually so.

2. Does the double or triple combination mentioned above have a therapeutic value of the same order as major endocrine surgery—adrenalectomy or hypophysectomy? On this point, too, there seems to be no conclusive evidence. Centers with a great deal of experience of endocrine surgery can claim very long remissions, 8—10 years or even longer. The series of hypophysectomies carried out at the In-

stitut Gustave-Roussy, which we describe below, also includes several remissions and survivals of this order, permitting in certain cases the patient's complete recovery and social reintegration. We have so far seen no proof that equal benefits derive from the use of drug combinations. This is why, in the present state of affairs, the Institut Gustave-Roussy reserves such treatment for cases where the destruction of the hypophysis by radioactive implantation is contraindicated.

3. There is also the question whether in the younger woman these drug combinations may not under certain circumstances aggravate the cancer, in the same way as estrogens given alone. It may well be that this is an idle fear, but we prefer to reserve this treatment for women over 50 years of age.

4. It is, however, certain that the relative proportions of the two or three hormones most frequently used in combination have been determined in a thoroughly empirical manner. It would be interesting to know whether different proportions would give better results.

5. There is an equal amount of uncertainty about the type of lesion which can profit from this treatment. Lesions of the soft tissues would appear to constitute the major indication.

I. Direct Action on the Endocrine Glands

The simplest and most frequently used example of the destruction of an endocrine tissue is that of the ovaries, whether surgical or radiological. We shall explain the indications below. On the other hand, the question of choice of technique for the suppression of ovarian function has been the subject of a special report from this Institute [40].

Castration may be effected in two ways: by oophorectomy or by irradiation. In our early period we tended to favor oophorectomy as being safer and more effective. Later on we re-examined our preference for surgical treatment in the light of the difficulty of persuading patients recovering from a mastectomy to undergo a further operation, and of the apparently satisfactory results obtained by other authors by means of radiological castration. Finally, to enable us to base our choice on objective criteria, we carried out a statistically controlled biological trial of the two methods: irradiation of the ovaries and bilateral oophorectomy.

1. Biological Comparison of Oophorectomy and Ovarian Irradiation

It would have taken too long to test the two methods for their influence on the development of the cancer. We therefore decided to use as our criterion of comparison the amount of gonadotrophins (HGH or GPH) excreted in the urine. The amount is greatest when estrogen production is low, thus when the suppression of ovarian function is most complete.

The technique of measuring the gonadotrophins and the statistical analysis of the results have been the subject of another paper [40]. We shall simply note here that it was the surgical patients who were included in this study. They were allocated at random to two groups: one group comprised patients born in a year ending in an odd number—these were castrated by irradiation (19 cases); the other group were born in a year ending in an even number (15 cases)—these were castrated by surgery. The 24-hour urinary excretion of gonadotrophins was measured 2 and 6 months after castration. Suitably diluted fractions of this urine were injected into immature mice. The gonadotrophin content was assessed on the the basis of the weight of the uterine horns of these animals.

Table 28. *Comparison of average weight (mg) of uterine horns of mice injected with urine of patients castrated by surgical or radiological methods at 2 and 6 months after castration*

Time after castration	Method	Dilution 1/200	1/100	1/50	1/25
2 mo.	Surg.	7.5	12.9	16.7	21.3
	Rad.	8.7	12.4	17.2	22.4
	(S < 0.05)	No	No	No	No
6 mo.	Surg.	8	9.9	13.5	20
	Rad.	8.3	14.3	19.5	23.1
	(S < 0.05)	No	Yes	Yes	No

There is very little to choose between the two methods—radiotherapy or surgery. After 2 months there is no statistically significant difference in gonadotrophin titers. After 6 months, however, there is an advantage in favor of irradiation, at least, at 2 out of the 4 dilutions (1/100 and 1/50) tested. It looks as if between the second and the sixth months the level of gonadotrophins continues to rise in irradiated patients, while it tends to fall in oophorectomized patients. In other words, estrogen depression seems to be deeper and longer-lasting after irradiation than after surgery. If we can have confidence in the method of measuring gonadotrophins practised by our group, this experiment shows that the radiological method is preferable to surgery. This result, which at first sight seems paradoxical, is hard to explain. There are two possible hypotheses.

The first is based on the postulated existence in some women of accessory ovarian tissue, situated within the pelvis but outside the ovaries proper; if this tissue were to remain following surgery, it could re-establish ovarian function after oophorectomy, whereas it would be rendered inactive by total irradiation of the pelvis. We could also invoke the presence of aberrant adrenal tissue situated in the pelvis, which is also irradiated at the same time as the ovaries.

The second hypothesis is more questionable: it postulates the selectivity of ovarian irradiation; indeed, this is carried out at doses which, while effectively preventing the follicles from developing into maturity, spares the other parts of the ovary. These may have some part to play in the equilibrium existing between the ovary and the other endocrine glands, such as the hypophysis or the adrenals. Since the action of the radiation is only upon some cells, sparing the rest of the ovary and its connective tissues, its anatomical selectivity would be reflected at the physiological level, where it would be concentrated on the elimination of estrogens. On the other hand, the suppression of the whole of the ovarian tissue and the rupture of its connections by oophorectomy would bring about non-selective disturbances. Moreover, the physiological disturbances created by oophorectomy are more immediately and deeply felt than those associated with irradiation and they provoke a hormonal deficit which one might at first believe to be total. For this reason, they may be able to stimulate earlier and more pronounced compensatory processes in other glands, such as the adrenal. The response to the two methods may thus be even more divergent when the time factor is taken into account: the action of surgery being not only total, but more

Table 29. *Surgical castration: frequency and 5-yr survival of patients with breast cancer + ovarian metastases*

Category	Total	Initial surgery	Surgery after radiotherapy	Surgery impossible	Treated before referral to IGR
Total castrated	148	52	47	17	32
% with ovarian metastases	11	8	6	12	22
% of total with ovarian metastases presumed cured after 5 years	1.3	2	2	0	0

immediate, and the action of irradiation being not only selective but also progressive and more physiological.

The deficiencies of these hypotheses are clear enough. We must hope that fresh work will be done to explain the mechanisms involved and their chronology.

Whatever these may turn out to be, the fact remains that in our comparative study irradiation of the ovaries produced a more complete suppression of estrogen impregnation than did bilateral oophorectomy. Furthermore, this finding is not really as paradoxical as it appears at first sight. Some earlier work has already queried the superiority of oophorectomy, in particular the very interesting study by DICSFALUZY et al. [10]. These authors first irradiated the ovaries of 17 women; five months later they performed an oophorectomy on the same patients. Measurements of estrogen excretion showed that the reduction in estrogen production caused by irradiation was not significantly enhanced by the excision of the ovaries. In fact, the latter appeared incapable of improving upon the prior irradiation. Objectively, therefore, we have two studies carried out by completely different methods and based on different tests, but whose conclusions agree in recognizing that castration by irradiation has a biological efficacy at least equal to and probably better than that of surgical castration.

2. Irradiation of the Ovaries Versus Oophorectomy

The factors involved in the choice between surgical castration and castration by irradiation may now be reviewed:

a) on the biological level—two studies, one [10] based on the measurement of estrogens and the other (I G-R) on that of gonadotrophins, indicating that irradiation is at least as effective as surgery;

b) on the carcinological level—no proof has been supplied of the superiority of either method;

4*

c) on the clinical level—in the absence of objective data and despite the reservations made above, the only convincing argument at present is that radiotherapy is a simple means of effecting castration and, in any case, simpler than surgery.

It must indeed be admitted that irradiation causes only slight discomfort to the patient. For those who require post-operative regional radiotherapy, the five or six sessions on the ovaries are easily fitted into the course of treatment. As for those being treated for castration only, the three or four sessions are always carried out in less than a week on an out-patient basis. Thus, the inconvenience of attending several times at the hospital is very much less than that of having to be admitted for several days for a surgical operation. This social advantage is matched by a considerable financial advantage, since irradiation is much cheaper.

It was finally this argument of convenience which persuaded us for several years now at the Institut Gustave-Roussy to give preference to ovarian irradiation, since the biological, carcinological and clinical tests have so far been unable to prove the superiority of one method over the other. If proof is eventually forthcoming in favor of surgery, we would, of course, revise our position.

We have to consider in particular the circumstances of the indication for castration. Systematic castration, carried out on symptomless patients, is well served by the delayed action of irradiation. On the other hand, when therapeutic castration has to be carried out on patients with a developing cancer, there are certain problems. It may indeed appear more advantageous to obtain a rapid action because the lesions are already extensive and because the cancer is rapidly growing, and, above all, because it is painful, as with bone metastases. Although there are no valid indications regarding the movement of the hormonal level in the days immediately following one or the other method of castration, and although we have known spectacular results to follow irradiation under these conditions, it does seem that in these particular cases oophorectomy, with its earlier and more abrupt effect is to be preferred. Thus, we recommend surgery whenever the patient's condition is such as to demand an immediate effect.

Furthermore, we have also to consider patients presenting with an associated gynecological disorder, such as an uterine or ovarian tumor. In such cases we always consult the gynecologist, and where these gynecological lesions require surgery, simultaneous oophorectomy is requested.

Apart from these two special situations—need for immediate action, or an associated gynecological condition requiring surgery in any case—candidates for castration are treated by irradiation at the Institut Gustave-Roussy.

The beneficial action of castration being a recognized fact appearing to arise from the removal of organic estrogens, it seemed to Huggins [11] that the failures of this method, or its reduced efficacy, could be the result of persisting estrogen production by the adrenals. This hypothesis has inspired trials with bilateral adrenalectomy in an attempt to remove this additional source of estrogen.

3. Hypophysectomy

Hypophysectomy has the same physiological justification as oophorectomy, inasmuch as the production of adrenal estrogens is controlled by the secretion of ACTH. It has in addition a triple theoretical advantage:

a) it permits the inhibition not only of the main adrenal glands but also of the accessory ones which exist in at least 50% of subjects and which, being of uncertain location, cannot be surgically excised;

b) it removes the source of prolactin and growth hormone as well as ACTH, and there is reason to suppose that these also stimulate the development of breast cancer;

c) it does not interfere with the secretion of aldosterone. Thus hypophysectomized patients are less disabled than those who have undergone adrenalectomy.

These are established facts concerning major endocrine surgery, but they take into account only some of its therapeutic effects.

The longer the interval between mastectomy and the first evidence of metastasis, the greater the importance of androgen secretion, and therefore the greater are the chances of success. Moreover, the therapeutic success of prior castration frequently augurs the success of more extensive endocrine surgery.

Finally, this is a treatment which can only be given to patients in a relatively well-preserved state of health.

Major endocrine surgery is relatively traumatic. We do not refer here to the risks of the operation, which are now minimal when it is carried out by an experienced team and the indications for operation have been properly interpreted. The problems arise mainly in the psychological field. The patients in question are often women who have been maimed by their disease and by the numerous therapeutic procedures to which they have been exposed. It is often difficult to persuade them to agree to bilateral lombotomy or fronto-parietal craniotomy. What is more, the doctor advising them often lacks the conviction to persuade them to accept a drastic treatment offering a bare 50% chance of success.

For these reasons, we at the Institut Gustave-Roussy have deliberately chosen to effect destruction of the pituitary function by yttrium-90 implantation. After an experience of 10 years and more than 300 cases, we have one of the longest series of this type in the world [63].

The stereotaxic technique of intrahypophyseal yttrium implantation used at the Institut Gustave-Roussy is, with a few minor differences, substantially that described by TALAIRACH in 1956 [7].

In the succeeding 8 years there have been various modifications aimed at increasing the safety, reducing the complications and multiplying the number of total pituitary destructions. We shall not go into the technical details of this method, which have been published elsewhere [32]. We have, however, in a good many cases been able to reduce the incidence of major complications of the operation by the use of technical modifications (use of non-radioactive peripheral grains, systematic implantation of yttrium grains in the sella turcica, terminal paraffinization).

The main features are the following:

1. although the operation requires a general anesthetic, operative trauma is minimal;

2. psychological trauma is equally slight. When the transnarinal technique is used, the operation leaves no visible scar. For this reason, it is often easier to obtain the patient's consent;

3. the daily chores which accompany any hypophysectomy include the administration of steroids and thyroid extracts. Moreover, diabetes insipidus, frequently

transitory, is often seen, requiring the additional administration of post-hypophyseal extracts;

4. its physiological results have been much improved by the adoption of a number of technical modifications, also described elsewhere [41]. At present, the rate of complete hypophyseal destruction achieved is of the order of 75%;

5. its therapeutic results compare well with those attained by other methods of endocrine surgery. Of a total of 300 women receiving an yttrium-90 implantation, we have recorded 30% with objective remissions (assessed by the classic criteria: regression of lesions for longer than 3 months, or stabilization over a period of 6 months), and after 10 years we can claim one remission lasting $8^1/_2$ years, one of 7 years and seven of 4 years.

The results are particularly spectacular where there are painful bone metastases, attenuation or complete cessation of the pain being achieved in three-quarters of our cases. This relief of pain also occurs in many cases where, on strictly objective criteria, the operation must be accounted a failure. The mechanism of this pain-relieving effect is obscure. We have shown that it is independent of the mechanism of the braking of pituitary function which is what induces the regression of the cancerous lesions.

Long-lasting objective regressions are almost always the result of total destruction of the hypophysis. On the basis of the 24-h I^{131} uptake, which is a satisfactory method of evaluating the extent of physiological destruction of the hypophysis, an uptake of 15% or less reasonably suggests total hypophysectomy. We currently achieve this result in over 75% of patients.

Table 30. *Morbidity of first series of 300 treated by intrahypophyseal yttrium implantation at the IGR*

	All 300		First 100	Sec. 100	Third 100	Remarks
Paralysis of 2nd, 4th and 6th cranial pairs	9	(3%)	6	3	0	Unilateral in 8 out of 9 cases
Serious damage to optic nerves	6	(2%)	5	1	0	No case of total blindness; unilat. in 4 out of 6 cases
Fistulae of sellar floor (rhinorrhea)	25	(8%)	15	4	6	Persistence of fistula for 3 yrs treated by waxing sella turcica
Meningites	11	(4%)	6	2	3	
Diabetes insipidus	232	(77%)	79	77	76	

Table 31. *Mortality of series of 300 intrahypophyseal yttrium implantations*

	All 300	First 100	Sec. 100	Third 100	Remarks
Death within 48 h	6 (2%)	5	1	0	
Death within 1 mo.	18 (6%)	12	4	2	Of the 18 deaths, 11 were due to cancer, i. e. erroneous indications for operation

Even when carried out by an experienced team, yttrium-90 implantation is not a completely innocuous operation.

Tables 30 and 31, where the patients are grouped under consecutive 100s, show how the complications resulting from the operation became progressively fewer, with the exception of diabetes insipidus, which in most cases is easily managed.

Post-operative mortality followed the same regressive curve. As stated above, major surgery is not for the moribund. All deaths occurring in the period immediately following the operation, even though they may be caused by the cancer itself, must therefore be debited to the operation. As can be seen from Tables 31 and 32, such cases are now rare with us.

Summing up the main aspects and problems of this method:

1. When carried out by a team who take great care to obtain complete hypophysolysis (as opposed to inserting a few grains of radioactive material in the sella turcica at random), this method is capable of producing prolonged remissions of excellent quality. In most cases this remission has an undeniable human value and is not merely a more or less vegetative prolongation of life.

2. The nature of the relief of pain obtained in cases of painful bone metastases remains the chief mystery of this method. Only one thing is certain: contrary to conventional opinion, the inhibition of the hypophyseal-adrenal axis probably has nothing to do with it.

3. The essential problem lies in the position which yttrium-90-induced hypophysolysis should occupy in the treatment of extensive breast cancers. There is no question as to the value of the treatment, but even the successive improvements in the technique have not made it completely safe. However slight it may be, the risk of creating a fistula exists, and this opens the door to meningeal infection.

On the other hand, we are not completely convinced that any of the other methods described has an equal therapeutic value. Certainly combinations of estrogen and progestogen and of estrogen-progestogen-steroid are effective; but are they capable of bringing about such prolonged organic and functional improvement? We cannot yet answer this question. But in any case it seems doubtful whether, even if their therapeutic value is equal, one can persuade patients to continue to take hormones regularly over a period of many years, particularly when they are liable to cause side-effects.

The respective positions of hormone treatment by means of surgery or drugs is a problem which confronts us every day. For ourselves, at the stage where the lesions have gone beyond the extent that can be controlled by local/regional treatments, whether surgical or radiological, we tend to lean fairly heavily upon yttrium-90 implantation, reserving the combined drug therapy mentioned above for cases where hypophysolysis is contra-indicated, until such time as there is irrefutable proof of their therapeutic equivalence.

In conclusion, let us note that a study of 19 autopsies [56] on patients who had undergone this operation (18 of whom had breast cancer), showed the originality of the delayed manner in which the necrosed pituitary gland reacts. The special characteristics of its organization bring about a most unusual inflammatory reaction which does not involve the cells, being predominantly vascular. This type of reaction can be compared to inflammation of the serous membranes.

Further away from the hypophysis, the surrounding structures sometimes exhibit only very minimal microscopic lesions which have no clinical echo.

Finally, a study of patients who have had hypophysectomy showed that it can effect remarkable anatomical transformations, particularly as regards the suprarenal cortex, where atrophy or even complete disappearance of the reticular or fascicular tissues is observed, while the glomerular structure is invariably preserved. Moreover, in the most successful cases the invaded bone shows a clear tendency to repair lytic tumoral lesions by metamorphic ossification from the tumoral stroma upwards.

J. Chemotherapy

Advanced breast cancer responds fairly well to chemical treatments and, whatever the product used, we have over the years tried numerous variations of treatment, ringing the changes on the substances, the doses and their proportions.

Chemotherapeutic drugs act by disrupting the mitotic cycle at various of its phases. The death of the cells follows after a longer or shorter interval. This effect may be obtained in two ways: either by changing an essential element in cell division (generally a nucleic acid), or by inhibiting the synthesis of this element at various stages of its function in vivo.

1. Nitrogen Mustards

Alkylating agents are the main representatives of the first category. Those we have used most frequently in the treatment of breast cancer are nitrogen mustards:

a) Karyolysin, the total dose of which should not exceed 3 μg/m^2 in five days;

b) Endoxana—here the maximum dose is variable, ranging from 0.5 to 7 g/m^2 per week;

c) Degranol—not more than 0.75 g/m^2 per course of treatment;

d) derivatives of ethyleneimine, the best known of which is Thiotepa which, however, has the drawback of delayed toxicity, so that no single treatment should exceed a total dose of 75 μg/m^2 which must be given at intervals of at least one month.

2. Antimetabolites

In the second category (antimetabolites) we should mention:

a) an antifolic: Methotrexate (or Amethopterin) of which the total dose per treatment varies with different schedules, ranging from 4 μg/m^2 per day for five days to 75 μg/m^2 i. v. in a single dose, with or without citrovorum factor;

b) an antipyrimidine: 5-fluorouracil, of which the total dose may be 600 μg/m^2 daily.

The doses of these two substances vary considerably according to whether they are given as a slow perfusion or intravenously, the oral route being far less effective. Thus, Methotrexate injected in a continuous 24-hour perfusion shows signs of toxicity before a total of 30 μg/m^2 has been reached, if injected discontinuously, whereas intravenously double or treble this amount can be given without distress.

With 5-fluorouracil, the contrary is the case: when given i.v. in a short time it is toxic and not much over 30 g/m² can be administered, whereas 3 or 4 times this amount can be given in each course of treatment if it is administered by our perfusion technique, giving 250 µg/h for a daily dose of 15 mg/kg.

3. Products Whose Mechanism of Action Has Not Been Clearly Established

a) substances extracted from microorganisms, such as mytomycin, actinomycin and rubidomycin;

b) various synthetic substances such as methyl hydrazine, with a total dose of about 3 g/m² in 3 weeks.

The doses we have given for each of these substances are, of course, theoretical quantities and are dependent on individual susceptibility and on the fractions and spacing in which the doses are given. Thus, one must keep a careful watch for signs of toxicity which may occur early or late, and sometimes arise suddenly and abruptly a few days or even several weeks after the end of a treatment.

Apart from certain toxic effects specific to certain substances (polyneuritis with the vinca alkaloids, cardiac complications with rubidomycin), the secondary effects of chemotherapeutic agents appear most often in the digestive tract and in the hemopoietic organs. Hematological complications most frequently affect the three cell lines: platelets, leucocytes and erythrocytes, so that it is essential to obtain regular hemograms of patients receiving this treatment, 2 or 3 times a week at the start of a course, and to stop treatment as soon as the white cell count falls below 2000 and the platelets below 100,000. This further implies a very cautious approach to the treatment of patients with disseminated bone and medullary localizations.

Digestive troubles may range from simple nausea to persistent vomiting and diarrhea, or from simple stomatitis to gastric ulceration, so that there, too, careful supervision is essential.

Finally, a complication of lesser severity, but one which has a profound psychological effect on the patient: alopecia, which is most often seen after prolonged treatment with Endoxana.

All of these products have sometimes produced prolonged remissions, used either separately or in association, but such combinations are always carefully planned and include simultaneously substances whose impact on the cells is different. For instance, an antimetabolite combined with a spindle cell poison or an alkylating agent.

On the strength of past experience of chemotherapeutic treatment of our patients, we can make a certain number of statements which can serve as the foundation of future policy:

1. There is no difference in the susceptibility to chemical treatment of patients who formerly reacted favorably to hormone treatment and those who did not.

2. When a patient responds well to chemical treatment, this therapy should be continued until the disease starts to develop again, at which point an attempt should be made with another product or combination. There is a whole series of products whose mechanism of action has not been clearly established. They include:

3. We have often been able to control disease in a patient with a new drug when she had become resistant to one, two, even three and, on occasion, four earlier chemotherapeutic treatments.

Throughout the whole of the period 1960—1965, as new drugs made their appearance, some ephemerally, we were able to maintain over a period of several years a number of patients who developed resistance within 4—5 months, but for whom we were lucky enough to obtain new drugs for testing. Unfortunately, this is no longer the case today.

4. A last point which is very important in evaluating results is that patients presenting with multiple metastases, which is the usual fate of patients undergoing chemotherapy, have quite different reactions according to the localization. Thus, bone metastases, with rare exceptions, never seem to respond to chemotherapy and appear to be the exclusive realm of hormone treatment.

On the other hand, visceral metastases, and in particular hepatic metastases, react in a not insignificant number of cases to chemotherapy, especially to the antipyrimidines. 5-Fluorouracil seems to be the preferred treatment for metastases of the liver in breast cancer.

As regards local/regional pleural or pulmonary metastases, their sensitivity to chemotherapy is very variable, and it has happened that we have seen lymph-node metastases disappear and pulmonary metastases grow, or vice versa.

For all these reasons, it is very difficult to give any objective appreciation of the results of chemotherapy in treating breast cancer.

K. Immunotherapy

Immunotherapy has been discovered too recently to have passed into the repertoire of current clinical treatment, but its general principle is that the cancer cell is destroyed following the formation of antibodies by the host. The antibodies are humoral or cellular antibodies and are directed against the antigens belonging to the malignant cell.

Breast tumors seem to be one of the more hopeful indications for treatment by immunotherapy, for here the cancerous cell is distinguished from the normal cell, if not by the presence of a given antigen, at least by the fact that it is present in much greater numbers.

Indeed, some authors have described the presence of circulating antibodies in the serum of many patients with breast cancer. These antibodies, identified by immunofluorescence or by passive hemagglutination, react with a protein antigen, lactotransferrin, which is present in the cancerous tissues, in embryonic tissues, in colostrum, in milk and, to a much smaller extent, in the mammary gland. No-one has yet been able to demonstrate the exact role of these circulating antibodies, but they certainly provide evidence of the existence in some cases of a specific host-tumor reaction.

The ideal would be, before we start to use immunotherapy, that we should understand the reciprocal influences exerted by the tumor and the host's immunological defenses. To this end, we have carried out two types of study at the Institut Gustave-Roussy—static and dynamic [57].

The static study enabled a relationship to be established between the state of cellular immunity (as assessed by skin tests of delayed hypersensitivity to tuberculin), and invasion of the lymph nodes. The study covered 233 subjects, 82 of whom had benign lesions and 151 malignant tumors, and all of whom had undergone surgery. Their N+ or N— condition had been determined by a histological examination of lymph nodes removed during the operation, by the procedure used at the Institut Gustave-Roussy.

An analysis of the results (Table 32) shows a distinct difference between the behavior of the N+ subjects, who have very weak responses, and N— subjects whose reactions are statistically very similar to those of subjects with benign lesions.

Table 32. *Skin test and immune situation*

	No. of patients	Skin test			
		— No.	%	+ No.	%
Benign lesions	82	30	36.5	52	63.4
Malignant lesions	151	90	59.6	61	40.3
N—	53	21	39.6	32	60.3
N+	98	69	70.4	29	29.6

Should we assume that the modifications of the architecture of the lymph nodes are responsible for the loss of their biological functions?

In fact, the invasion is very often spotty and, although at present we have no formal argument to support this hypothesis, we think it much more likely that lymphatic invasion is favored by a prior weakening of immunity. Moreover, the manner of the development of the disease of cancer also seems, if not conditioned by, at any rate linked with the extension of lymph-node invasion. This is borne out by the second study of this problem carried out at the Institut Gustave-Roussy.

The dynamic study confirmed the gravity of the N+ forms, whose 3-year survival rate is definitely lower than that of the N— forms, but it also provided a supplementary piece of evidence: according to whether the lymph-node barrier is crossed or not, the dissemination of the cancerous process will follow different courses.

Recurrences in the N+ forms are most often manifested in a local/regional fashion, whereas in N— cases the extension of the disease is effected by the hematogenous route with distant visceral localizations.

Pulmonary metastases are seen with equal frequency in both categories (see Fig. 3, p. 19).

The explanation of facts like these is far from simple. In cases of lymphatic invasion, what are the respective roles of the host's defense reaction, dissection and irradiation of the systematic lymphatic territories?

Looked at from this angle, the immunotherapy of cancer of the breast should comprise two components whose aims are:

1. to preserve the lymph nodes as far as possible from surgical or radiological destruction where this is clearly useless (N—);

2. to stimulate the immune defenses of either the cellular or humoral type in cases where it is possible to predict that one or other of these functions is inadequate.

Combined Treatments

From all that has so far been said, it is clear that we have available a number of techniques belonging to different disciplines, and each patient will usually require a combination of several techniques. Any increase in the chance of cure is likely to arise from the combination of these treatments.

II. Team Work — the Committee

The multidisciplinary nature of the necessary therapeutic measures basically involves three people: a physician, insofar as he represents chemotherapy and hormone therapy, a surgeon and a radiologist, supported by a pathologist.

Logically the need arises for machinery to ensure that they are able to consult with each other before any part of the therapeutic program is put into effect, and to share the resulting work between them. It is this prior consultation following a joint examination of the patient which accounts for much of the progress which has been achieved in making better use of the means at our disposal. It was with the idea of taking this idea of shared decision-making among colleagues to its logical conclusion that what we call "Localization Committees" have been set up at the Institut Gustave-Roussy.

These Committees therefore are composed of four people, three of whom have a permanent function and must be present when the decision concerning the treatment program is taken (physician, surgeon and radiologist). Each Committee looks after all tumors in a given organ or region.

It seemed essential to base the work of each Committee on a document, so this was drawn up at the very beginning: we call it the Treatment Protocol. Such a document, which lays down the policy to be followed at the Institut Gustave-Roussy in the treatment of a given tumor, must always be the outcome of a general discussion involving right from the start all who will at any time be concerned with the implementation of the actions noted in the program of treatment. It is particularly important that this general discussion should be as wide-ranging as possible, because it is inevitable that some of the actions on the treatment program will have to be carried out by people who were not present at the decision-making meeting. Thus, the essential condition on which they accept the decision is that they would have beeen entitled to discuss the principle involved at the time when the joint decision was made regarding the action to be taken in this or that particular clinical condition.

Thanks to this understanding, the Committee's decisions are reached with a minimum of argument, and a particular policy will be followed for a certain time. This does not mean that any given protocol is rigid and unalterable. It will be subject to revision as new facts come to light, either within the Institut or from outside it, but the process which will bring about the modification must be the same as the original one. The change will be made only after a fresh discussion, comprising all those whom it may concern.

The Treatment Protocol which guides every Committee contains:

1. the clinical description of all possible manifestations of cancer at the particular site with which the Committee is concerned, classified by UICC's TNM system;

the various criteria are recorded on a punched card and handled by computer. No doubt this procedure introduces a greater degree of standardization into the examination;

2. the description of the various therapeutic media which are available;

3. the points on the basis of which the treatment plan will be drawn up; thus, against each of the clinical categories defined by the Protocol the ideal treatment is prescribed, listing the order in which surgeon, radiologist and physician should intervene, and the techniques to be applied.

This text was drawn up with the assistance of all the specialists concerned, criticized by the Committee which has the responsibility of implementing it, and finalized by consultation with the Technical Committee composed of the heads of all the service departments at the Institut.

The three medical members of the Committee have the task of receiving the patients, examining them, establishing the diagnosis and the clinical classification and determining the treatment plan on the basis of the Protocol, having due regard to any unforseen local conditions.

In addition, each in his own field is responsible for liaison between the Committee and the technical department whose representatives they are in respect of carrying out that part of the plan that devolves upon them. Finally, they are jointly responsible for supervising the patient for a period of at least 15 years, if the patient lives that long. They are also responsible for contacts and correspondence, both inside and outside the Institut. This is the most perfect expression of collective responsibility.

To return to one of the most important elements of this structure: the decision regarding treatment must be taken jointly for each patient by the representatives of the three specialties involved after they have first made a joint study of all the data which shed light on the diagnosis and the clinical condition of the patient. It should also be noted that each of the Committees set up to deal with a particular localization includes persons representing the various technical departments concerned. Thus, for example, all the techniques concerned with radiation elect one of their number, regardless of his or her position in the hierarchy, to represent "radiotherapy" on the Committee. This member, like those representing the other techniques, is entitled to full participation in the discussion of the treatment plan within the framework of the Protocol.

In committee, in fact, the hierarchy is largely ignored, because the radiologist, for instance, will be present, not in his capacity as department head or assistant, but in his capacity as delegate acting on behalf of all technicians employing radiation, and on equal terms with his medical and surgical colleagues. It is indeed indispensable, if it is desired to give full expression to the team idea which postulates equality of skills, that each skill should be presented, defended and applied without any particular skill playing a predominant role and imposing its will on the others.

There are countries where the surgeons run the show and it is left to the radiologists to do what the surgeons cannot or will not do. In other countries, the situation is reversed: when carcinology is mentioned it is primarily radiology which is meant and surgery is not generally considered in a concerted discussion. Such a practice has grave drawbacks as regards the actual treatment, the result being that whichever specialist is consulted first, instead of considering whether some other specialty could not do better than his own or, at least, do as well using simpler means, starts off by doing everything within his power, at whatever cost to the patient, only passing her on to another specialist when he considers he has done all he can. The consequence will therefore be that he undertakes more than he should.

It will be observed that the procedure we have been describing functions at two levels: a level of technical application and a level of decision. The decision-making level is at the very heart of carcinology. A man does not have to be a carcinologist to know how to operate on or irradiate a patient with a malignant tumor. On the other hand, to know *when* to do it, he has to be qualified to take part in the multi-disciplinary discussion from which the treatment plan will emerge, and he has to be aware of what goes on outside his own discipline before he can usefully discuss matters with colleagues representing the other techniques and be capable of supporting or rejecting the points raised in discussion.

This is a feature which is on the whole peculiar to cancer Institutes, for there are few diseases where there is the same need to apply a variety of techniques in a coordinated manner for the benefit of a single patient according to a plan of treatment which varies with each localization.

One of the criticisms made of this system is that it is "inhuman" because it is more difficult to establish a human contact between the patient and a group than with a single doctor. However, on the technical level such a system offers the optimum conditions for the patient to benefit from the best possible understanding between the various persons concerned with her treatment, hence from the possibilities of choice of technique which will be best for her while being also the simplest available.

It is equally clear that since no single specialist or doctor can direct the complete treatment of such a patient from start to finish, we were forced to find a formula which, while maintaining the necessary personal contact between the patient and those who care for her, does not allow this contact to be transformed into a private domain from which all others are excluded.

Thus, for example, a general carcinologist who by force of circumstance finds himself acting as an intermediary between the patient and the cancer center, may have no share in her treatment because of the localization of the patient's disease: he will not be operating, because he is not a surgeon, nor irradiating her, because he is not a radiologist. He cannot, therefore, claim her as his property. Many doctors use the singular form of the personal possessive—"my" patient, whereas in a cancer center a patient can never be anything other than "our" patient.

Neither the techniques nor the procedures are inhuman; it is the men applying them who show more or less humanity. In each individual case it is easy enough, if it is really wanted, to arrange for each patient to have a mentor in the committee, proposed by its members and chosen by her as, so to speak, her advocate with the group. This appointment is not automatic but depends on the actual conditions of treatment. Let us suppose, for example, that the patient will be treated mainly by the surgeon and that the radiologist will have only a small part to play; then quite naturally the surgeon will become the patient's personal "advocate".

When the intermediary between the group and the patient is a member of the staff of the Institut, he retains this role of intermediary. The Committee sees to it that the intermediary

1. is regularly kept informed of progress;

2. shares in the establishment of the treatment plan, if he is able and wishes to;

3. if he so desires, he takes charge of correspondence with the private doctor outside the Institut.

Within the framework of these various conditions peculiar to cancer Institutes, and which are incompatible with a single doctor having a monopoly, there is plenty of room for the humanity of our work to make itself felt. The testimony of many different patients shows how satisfied they are with the technical side of the organization which gives them the feeling that each doctor has been able to make his own contribution, the end result being a coordinated plan. Thus, they are not pushed around from one person to another without any prior consultation.

III. The Treatment Protocol — its Various Parts

We have explained the factors whose value in the choice of a treatment policy can be judged by the work carried out at the Institut Gustave-Roussy; now we want to explain the factors of this policy which are applied in the construction of the Protocol used by the Committee for malignant tumors of the breast.

A. The T N M Classification

This is a system which enables each patient to be characterized on the basis of the clinical extension of the malignant lesion. The following are the aims of UICC's [3] T N M system for describing the clinical extension of malignant tumors.

1. To enable, before any treatment is given, a proper choice of therapy to be made by providing the means to define the clinical extension so that patients with similar extensions can be grouped together.

2. Hence to enable different institutions to speak the same language when communicating facts about what sort of patient receives what sort of treatment.

3. This again should enable comparisons to be made of the results obtained by these institutions on patients in the same clinical group who may be receiving different treatments.

4. It should offer the possibility of even greater precision with a view to aiding the choice of treatment, by refining the criteria by means of which patients are placed in one category rather than another. Retrospective research on the prognostic significance of the criteria used is one of the means by which the groups can be more precisely defined. Therefore it is not the main object of the T N M system to provide prognostic indicators.

5. It should leave room for any additional criteria, short of modifiying the initial definition, which can be used to supplement it, such as sex, age, histological status, etc. etc.

The letters T N M designate:

T = the clinical extension of the primary tumor
N = the clinical appearance of the adenopathy
M = the existence or not of distant metastases.

Each category is subdivided into: T1, T2 . . . , N0, N1 etc.
The strength of the T N M system is that it provides a descriptive system based on purely clinical signs which in no way excludes supplementary data.

---

[3] Union Internationale Contre le Cancer — International Union Against Cancer.

The problem is to *describe* an extension of the disease of cancer on the basis of clinical findings without falling into the trap of trying to interpret them, i. e. trying to attribute some significance to the findings.

The TNM system is, in fact, a sort of shorthand for characterizing a particular tumor. When the content of T1, T2 etc. was decided, every effort was made to define those features of the tumor which make it possible to distinguish the points that separate T1 from T2, T2 from T3 and so on.

It is clear that the "Union Internationale Contre le Cancer," wishing to create a common international language, must take the view that its proposed definitions of the various degrees of T, N and M must be recognized as UICC's property, a sort of "appellation contrôlée," in other words that the letters T, N, M should not be used other than for the definitions proposed by UICC. If anyone wishes to apply the basic principles of the system with different definitions of T, N and M, he is welcome to do so, but in this case he must use a different set of letters as well, and not TNM. If this rule were not observed, there would be a risk that two articles, using the letters TNM with different meanings, might be published in the same journal. Thus, if their meaning is not standardized, the system would create confusion instead of aiding comparison.

The Three Factors

It is now necessary to say a few words about each of these three factors and the principles applied in describing them.

1. T — the Primitive Tumor

The increasing degrees of extension of the primary tumor are indicated by the accompanying number. A selection of precisely definable characteristics or parameters must be made, exactly evaluated during the clinical examination and allocated precise limits, such as a range of dimension or a yes/no answer to a question like: Is it mobile or fixed?

Without doubt, the clinical observations on the patient should always include as many physical signs as possible, but it is neither necessary nor practicable to include them all in the definitions of the various categories of T. The choice must be made on the basis of physical signs, for example, the fixation of the breast tumor to the superficial pectoral aponeurosis. If two physical signs are normally found together, it is not necessary to mention them both and it is better to select the one which is more readily determined.

Example: two degrees of T are separated by skin fixation, or the absence of this sign.

Apart from the four degrees of T necessary to describe the extension of the tumor, there are various other symbols which should be mentioned. T0 means that no tumor can be detected clinically. This is the case, for example, where there is a bloody discharge from the nipple. It is necessary to have this category for cases where metastases arise through the lymph or blood circulation, while the primary tumor remains hidden.

These degrees represent particular situations—physical facts. Those who would like an essential feature of the system to be that each degree represents a different and rising level of severity are confusing the description with the possible consequences. What the TNM system tries to do by the addition of a number to the T or N is to describe groups of facts. The severity of the degrees may be different, but it will, in fact, depend on the treatment which is being given. What is the most serious today may well be the least serious tomorrow, whereas a characteristic like skin fixation is observed and recorded once and for all. The first objective of characterizing the individual categories of extension is to facilitate the choice of treatment and to enable hospitals to communicate with one another in terms that all can understand when describing cases receiving such-and-such a treatment.

Example: in one hospital cases without skin fixation are operated while those with skin fixation are not; in another they operate on both categories, while in a third they do not operate on either. However, both categories must be kept separate, otherwise the three hospitals will never be able to compare their results.

2. N — the Regional Lymph Nodes

The clinical observations regarding the lymph nodes are also expressed by a number, assessed independently from that for the primary tumor. N0 means that there is no palpable lymph node; N1, N2 etc. stand for the clinical finding of palpable adenopathies. In regions where it is impossible to examine the local lymph nodes, the term NX is used (obese patients or those who have had an axillary adenectomy before referral to the center).

The classification is conceived so as to be adaptable for particular localizations. According to the TNM rules, the "regional" lymph nodes of the breast are those of the axilla and supra- and infraclavicular regions. The question of the "significance" of adenopathies is a controversial one. Does the clinician consider a lymph node metastatic or not? The axillary region is a particularly good example. Leaving aside the arguments for or against "significance," we may assume that many doctors who judge an adenopathy on this basis are likely to be wrong as often as they are right. In every case where the lymph nodes are palpable, they should be classed as N1. If it is considered that they do not contain metastases, the category N1(a) may be used; if it is thought that they do, then N1(b).

To illustrate the use of the N categories in the classification of breast tumors, we have collected the data reported in Table 33.

Table 33. *Malignant breast tumors / Axillary lymph nodes*
T N M clinical N and histological N

		No. of cases	% N−	% N+
T1	N0	5	—	—
	N1	22	63%	37%
T2	N0	78	55%	45%
	N1	263	33%	67%
T3	N0	24	29%	71%
	N1	171	25%	75%
T4	N0	0	—	—
	N1	19	15%	85%

This table allows a comparison to be made between the clinical situation according to N0 or N1, which is a fact in itself, and the histological situation, which is also a fact. As can be seen from the table, if there is a relationship, it varies according to T. This is a good example of the use of separate criteria. No use has been made in this table of the possibility of introducing an intermediate category between the clinical assessment N1 and the histological subdivision N— or N+:

> N1(a) nodes not considered to contain growth
> N1(b) nodes considered to contain growth

as this addition is purely subjective. Table 33 gives an idea of the magnitude of the divergences and variations with T, quite apart from the clinical skill of the doctor who makes the classification.

The TNM system leaves open the possibility of introducing the results of the histological examination of surgically excised lymph nodes. Nobody can deny the significance of lymph node invasion, although, as we have shown, the confirmation of such invasion depends very much upon the care devoted to the examination. The symbols + (plus) and — (minus) are then added.

Example: a lymph node is mobile (N1): at this stage of the description it is impossible to say more. To try to guess whether a node is invaded or not is simply to make a random interpretation. If one of the techniques applied during treatment provides additional information, this may be added as a supplement, but it cannot be allowed to modify the initial clinical category.

Example: if the patient in the preceding example is operated upon, the surgeon when he examines the N1 lymph node will know for certain whether it is N+ or N—. In this case, he will add + or — to the N1, hence N1+ or N1—, the important point being that the case will still be labelled N1, since this allows it to be compared with other N1 cases which have not been operated.

To take another example, the histological condition of the lymph nodes will be given as NX+ or NX—, because they were not clinically accessible (NX) but examined histologically after the operation.

3. M — Distant Metastases

The absence or presence of metastases is indicated by the letter M. M0 means that the clinical examination was negative and M1 that a metastasis exists, other than in the regional lymph nodes, at the time when the patient is first seen. M1 can be subdivided into sub-categories to indicate the type of metastasis, e. g. bone, liver, lungs etc. Obviously, the clinical detection of metastases will depend upon the available equipment and will vary from one hospital to another. Radiographs of the thorax, spine and pelvis would appear essential in breast cancer patients.

We should note that any findings that can be derived from a mammography are not included in the TNM system, the reason for this being that this was considered premature; its potentialities and correct interpretation were not thought to be sufficiently widely understood. However, if this situation were one day to change, there would be nothing against including it. The TNM system is open to all improvements.

To sum up, TNM is an analytical descriptive notation, composed of criteria with successive subdivisions, and allowing new data to be incorporated without modifying the existing notation. It also enables all other existing or future criteria—age, sex, site, histological appearance—to be placed in parallel without modifying the annotations already made, which remain permanently on record for subsequent analysis.

The T N M system is based on the description, before treatment of any kind is given, of the extent of three major facets of the malignant process which are recorded separately and may, if so desired, be analysed separately. Such studies have been made, particularly at the Institut Gustave-Roussy [42]. There is no doubt they will be made more frequently in future.

Both staging and classification by T N M degrees show the progress of the development of the disease. Both methods have certain limitations. If we consider malignant breast tumors, for which four stages are provided, it is necessary to define the limits of each stage. On the whole, agreement on stages I and IV is easy, the former representing a well-localized attack, and the latter a stage where metastases are widespread. It is the intermediate stages II and III which are most difficult to define and about which clinicians are seldom unanimous. Stage III, in particular, is often very broad and includes patients whose survival time will have a very wide scatter according to the extension of the disease. Hence it is often necessary to subdivide these stages thereby, of course, increasing their number. In practice, therefore, four stages are not enough, but are there perhaps too many possible T N M groups? If we take breast cancer, for which there are provided 4 degrees of T, 4 degrees of N and 2 degrees of M, giving a total of 32 possible combinations, it must be conceded that this is so.

McKay and Sellers [43], analysing 1219 cases of breast cancer, found that two of the 32 groups did not contain a single patient, and that 12 contained less than 10 cases. This problem deserves closer study, but all the same it is clear that it is better to have a large number of T N M groups, which can be retrospectively combined into "new" stages in the light of experience without the need to modify in any way the initial description of the patient's disease, rather than to place patients once for all the first time they are seen into stages which are over-rigidly defined and cannot be changed without modifying the definitions of the degrees of extension.

Definitions of T, N and M for Malignant Breast Tumors

The code number for breast cancer in the International Classification of Diseases (1955) is 170. The UICC Committee has proposed the following anatomical divisions for the breast:

170.1 — Medial half
0.2 — Lateral half
0.3 — Sub-areolar
0.4 — Other
0.5 — Not stated

T N M Category of Malignant Breast Tumors

The following definition of the T N M categories is proposed for the breast:

T Primary Tumor

T0   No evidence of primary tumor.
T1   Tumor 2 cm or less in greatest dimension.
     Skin not involved, except in the case of Paget's disease confined to nipple.
     No retraction of nipple.
     No pectoral muscle fixation.
     No chest wall fixation.
T2   Tumor more than 2 cm but not more than 5 cm in greatest dimension, or
     incomplete skin fixation (tethered or dimpled), or
     nipple retraction (in subareolar tumors), or
     Paget's disease extending beyond the nipple.
     No pectoral muscle fixation.
     No chest wall fixation.
T3   Tumor more than 5 cm but not more than 10 cm in greatest dimension, or skin
     fixation complete (infiltration or ulcerated), or
     peau d'orange in tumor area, or
     pectoral muscle fixation [4] (incomplete or complete).
     No chest wall fixation.
T4   Tumor more than 10 cm in greatest dimension, or skin involvement or peau
     d'orange wide of tumor but not beyond breast area, or chest wall fixation [5].

N Regional Lymph Nodes

The clinician may record whether palpable nodes are considered to contain growth or not.

N0   No palpable homolateral axillary nodes.
N1   Movable homolateral axillary nodes.
     N1a Nodes not considered to contain growth.
     N1b Nodes considered to contain growth.
N2   Homolateral axillary nodes fixed to one another or to other structures.
N3   Homolateral supra- or infra-clavicular nodes, movable or fixed, or edema of the arm [6].

M Distant Metastases

M0   No evidence of distant metastases.
M1   Distant metastases present.
     M1a   Skin involvement wide of breast.
     M1b   Involvement of contralateral nodes or contralateral breast.
     M1c   Clinical or radiographic evidence of metastases to lungs, pleural cavity,
           skeleton, liver, etc.

We have adopted this clinical classification in its entirety.

---

[4] Incomplete pectoral muscle fixation indicates that contraction of the muscle limits tumor mobility. Complete pectoral muscle fixation indicates that contraction of the muscle abolishes tumor mobility.

[5] The chest wall includes the ribs, intercostal muscles and serratus anterior muscle but not the pectoral muscle.

[6] Edema of the arm may be caused by lymphatic obstruction; lymph nodes may not then be palpable.

B. The Therapeutic Categories (Fig. 17)

The T N M classification is thus applied to every case which comes before the Committee; this is one of its essential functions because this classification, by the terms of the Protocol itself, will form the basis of the therapeutic indications.

We have distinguished the various criteria which form the basis of the T N M classification, so that we can proceed to a particular grouping, in the form of *Therapeutic Categories* whose composition will be more readily understood by reference to Fig. 17. This diagram shows all the factors of the TNM classification and allows our grouping to be easily understood. On the left are the four possibilities for T and, reading from left to right in 6 columns, the various criteria which define the different T categories; still further to the right are the factors which characterize the clinical appearance of the lymph nodes, as well as the presence or absence of distant metastases, completed by the presence or absence of the developing phase.

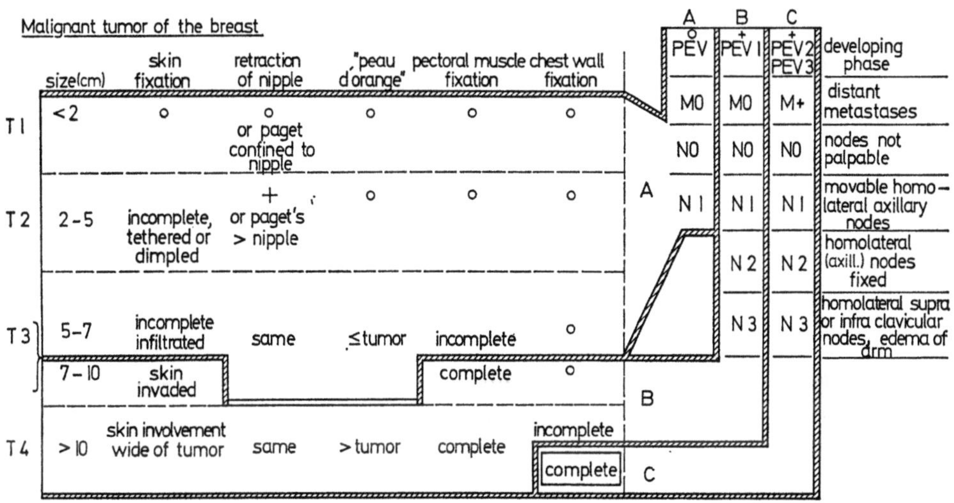

N.B. Category A patients with PEV I are transferred to category B

Fig. 17. *Therapeutic category according to TNM classification*

1. Category A

T1 and T2 are included in Category A. As regards T3, we have divided it according to the following criteria:

size — up to 7 cm in diameter in Category A;

fixation to skin — when there is incomplete fixation or infiltration, it belongs in Category A, but when the skin is invaded, the case goes into Category B;

retraction of the nipple and "peau d'orange"—no comment.

There is a further division as regards *fixation* to the *pectoralis major*. When, in the course of Tillaux mobilization, the contraction of the muscle merely restricts mobility, the case remains in Category A, but when the tumor is fixed by this process, the case goes into Category B.

The importance of this last distinction will be apparent when it is made clear that it corresponds to an important choice of therapy. This is where it is useful to have several doctors examining the patient to decide on the classification, as the presence of the radiotherapist and the surgeon, whose interests may differ, will certainly produce a classification closer to the real situation if they have differing opinions.

As regards the clinical appearance of the lymph nodes, classification is simple: forms without palpable nodes, or where the nodes are palpable but mobile, go into Category A. In addition, there must be no developing phase and no distant metastases perceptible.

2. Category B

If we look at Fig. 17, we see that Category B comprises:
tumors over 7 cm where the skin is involved
with peau d'orange extending beyond the tumor
with complete fixation to the pectoral muscle
with incomplete chest wall fixation (subdivision of T4).

All possible forms of N are included here. No distant metastases.
Forms in the PEV1 developing phase, if they have otherwise all the criteria for Category A, are transferred to Category B, or stay in it if they combine all the criteria for Category B.

3. Category C

This is characterized by three factors:
complete chest wall fixation
existence of distant metastases
or existence of PEV3 developing phase.

These are the three therapeutic categories as constituted on the basis of the TNM classification. The TNM details are preserved within each category so as to leave open the possibility of recombining different groups, if necessary, in order to make comparative studies. One of the built-in advantages of the TNM classification is that it allows subsequent recombinations to be made in the light of problems which may arise later on for clinicians and therapists.

C. Techniques

The Protocol includes a section which very broadly defines the techniques to be used by determining their limits, but naturally leaves it to each technical department to work out the details.

As we have already described the technical aspects of the procedures at the Institut Gustave-Roussy, we shall not repeat them here.

D. Therapeutic Indications (Fig. 18)

The Treatment Protocol is established for the three clinical categories defined above as follows.

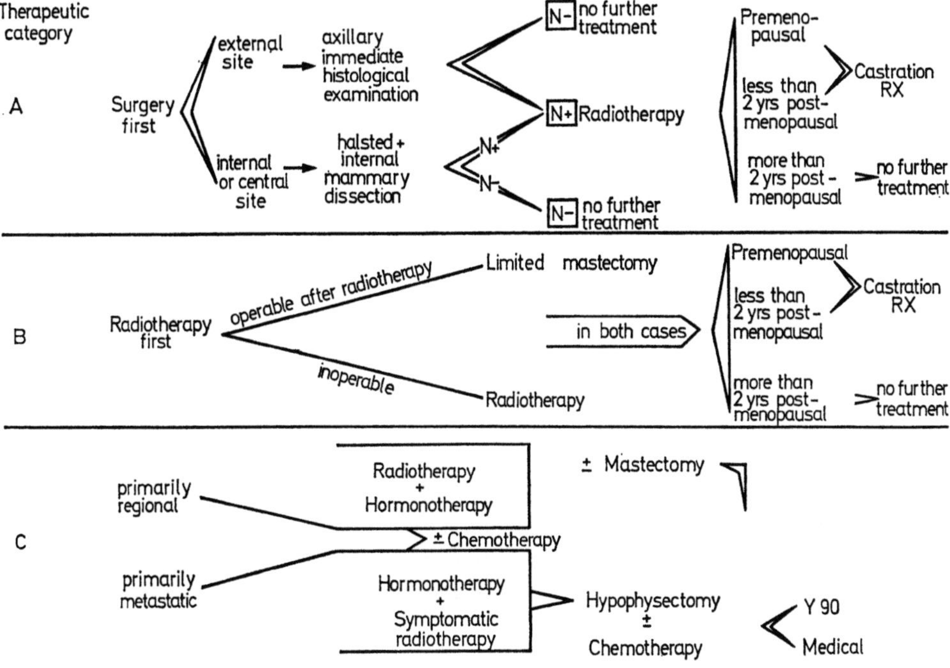

Fig. 18. *Therapeutic indications*

1. Category A

1st Period — Surgery

The cases which fall into this category are initially operable, but the surgical approach will differ according to the location of the tumor.

Tumors in the external quadrants. If the frozen-section histological examination of the tumor is positive, the frozen-section examination of the axillary lymph nodes follows immediately. The surgical procedure is completed according to the outcome of this examination: if $N-$, simple mastectomy, supplemented by axillary dissection; if $N+$, radical mastectomy (Halsted) plus internal mammary dissection.

Tumors which are central or in the internal quadrants. Radical mastectomy and internal mammary dissection. However, if the biopsy of the lymph nodes located next to the axillary vein, or of those found at the level of the first intercostal space shows them to be $N+$, internal mammary dissection is not carried out.

2nd Period — as Required, Radiotherapy or No Radiotherapy

Whatever the site of the tumor, the next phase of the treatment will be conditioned by the presence or absence of histologically confirmed metastases of the lymph nodes. If $N-$, *no radiotherapy* because, as we stated on p. 19, we consider there to be no risk of future regional recurrences. The risk of further manifestations, though rare with $N-$, is in any case that they will arise somewhere else. In the present state of our knowledge there is nothing to show that post-operative regional radiotherapy would reduce the risk of distant metastases developing, since if they exist, some will already have been there for a more or less long period before the operation. Therefore, we do not give post-operative radiotherapy for N— cases with an external tumor site, even though we are unable to check up on the internal mammary lymph nodes. The reason for this, as already explained, is that on comparing the various studies of the distribution of N— and N+ in the axillary and internal mammary lymph node chains, we find that, for a tumor in an external site, if the *detailed* examination of the axillary specimen shows it to be N—, then the internal mammary chain is also N—.

If N+, *post-operative radiotherapy* is given to all patients.

When, for any reason at all, it has not been possible to carry out internal mammary dissection with a central or internal tumor, radiotherapy is done for safety's sake, even if the axillary nodes are N—, because doubt remains regarding the state of the internal mammary chain.

3rd Period — Supplementary for N + Cases Only and as a Function of Age

With premenopausal patients or those only 2 years postmenopausal: systematic *castration,* either surgical or by irradiation. We have already explained why we prefer radiation at the Institut Gustave-Roussy.

Patients more than 2 years past the menopause are not prescribed any additional hormone therapy.

To sum up: Category A receives a surgical treatment during the 1st period of action, which may be the only one. Extra treatment is required by the presence of N+; this will be radiotherapy, either alone or combined with hormone therapy as a function of the hormonal status. This logical progression will depend on that vital period constituted by the careful investigation of the histological invasion of the lymph nodes. If we possessed an indirect but reliable method of predicting the condition of N, we should limit the treatment for Category A N— to simple mastectomy.

As stated, in principle we do not give additional chemotherapy. Therapeutic trials are in progress to evaluate whether this might be justified, but so far we have had no evidence to support its use.

2. Category B

To recapitulate, this category also comprises patients who would have been in Category A had they not had in addition a developing growth (PEV 1).

1st Period, Radiotherapy for All Patients

The treatment (Fig. 18) systematically applies initial radiotherapy. The first version, which we used until 1959, began with a radiological treatment which we hoped would allow simple mastectomy with axillary dissection to be performed after a dose equal to about half the total dose to be given, the treatment being completed by giving the remainder post-operatively. But it sometimes happened that this program could not be carried out correctly, and in certain Category B forms surgical intervention turned out to be impossible because of local or general contraindications, or the patient's refusal due to the reduction of the tumor.

At present we are using a second version, comprising *initial total radiotherapy*, a 2nd period which is in principle surgical (whenever possible, limited surgical intervention: simple mastectomy with or without axillary dissection). Here castration is effected whether the patients are N+ or N−, but only with those who are still menstruating, or in whom the menopause occurred no more than two years before.

As with Category A, and for the same reason, we do not use any additional chemotherapy.

3. Category C

This category embraces two groups of patients whose therapeutic prospects are different (see Fig. 18), although there is no clear division between them.

a) The first group is *primarily regional.* The extension makes the possibility of complementary surgery most unlikely. *Regional irradiation* to a dose of 4500 rads is the treatment which will probably be given, but without excluding the possibility of additive interstitial limited radiotherapy at superdoses. A simple mastectomy with axillary removal is not necessarily excluded, if this becomes possible, but we do not envisage extensive surgery which could involve parietal resection.

The complementary hormone period will comprise 1. *castration,* as for Catogories A and B; 2. *estrogen* for those more than 2 years postmenopausal.

b) The second group is *primarily of patients with distant metastases.* Here the regional treatment is relegated to second place, although it may include radiation, particularly for bone metastases with one, or very few foci, and exceptionally surgery if required, say, for an ulcerated mobile breast. Here such indications are considered more from the point of view of the patient's comfort rather than solely as cancer treatment. Our efforts are directed first towards stabilizing or slowing down the generalization.

Hormone therapy, which is the most effective medium for this, thus assumes prime importance. Over and above the conventional treatments, such as castration or estrogen for the older woman, one should first of all consider using medical hypophysiolysis (Lyndiol, 2 tablets a day, plus cortancyl at a dose of 30 µg per day) in cancer cases where the wide initial dissemination makes nonsense of purely local or partial treatment.

Hypophysectomy by yttrium transplantation is not considered until two years after the primary tumor has been treated or metastases have appeared. We have already discussed the appropriate conditions.

The *chemotherapy* of mammary carcinoma is not yet fully codified [55]. It can be very useful, particularly for localizations in the soft tissues and visceral parts. Remissions are sometimes achieved by this means but, with the analytical factors at present available to us, it is impossible to predict where they will be effective.

We prefer to use two formulas:

Formula A: 5-fluorouracil perfused daily
Thiotepa in 10-day series (max. 10 µg daily) given through the perfusion tube at 4-week intervals.

A check must be made for diarrhea (5-fluorouracil) and on platelets and white cells (Thiotepa). The toxicity of the latter is delayed for 3 weeks.

Formula B: Methotrexate injected subcutaneously at a rate of 2.5 µg every 6 h
for 6 or 7 days, followed by one third of this dose once a month.
Check platelets.

With postmenopausal patients over 55 years of age, estrogens and progestogens may
have a beneficial effect on the tumor or on cutaneous lesions.

Generally speaking, local treatment assumes secondary importance once generalization has been confirmed. However, lymph-node metastases, distal or cutaneous
metastases, and some isolated bone metastases, should not definitely contraindicate
regional treatment. Not infrequently, it takes years for the disease to attain its full
extent. It would therefore be a mistake not to try to stabilize it at the level of the
breast or the adjacent lymphatic areas, if for no other reason than to improve the
patient's physical and psychological well-being. Cancers which show a reduced
activity (squirrhous carcinoma), or which are brought before the doctor at a late
stage because they have developed so slowly, should be treated energetically; this is
where radiotherapy and simple mastectomy find their true place.

It is impossible to mention all the clinical eventualities which may arise under
Category C, as there are too many combinations of the various types of regional
lesions with distant metastases.

As regards bone metastases, if castration is not effective in relieving pain, or if
there are functional risks connected, for example, with the likelihood of a fracture,
radiation is employed.

A similar type of irradiation is also suited to the treatment of distal or broncho-
pulmonary lymph-node lesions, even when they are isolated. The same indication is
valid for cerebral metastases, although here it is more questionable. However, irradiation of the entire content of the cranium sometimes produces unexpected remissions, but clearly it must be reserved for specially selected cases. Attempts to treat
liver metastases by irradiation have been very disappointing, and where these are
present we do not go beyond a symptomatic treatment or chemotherapy (5 Fu).

We should also mention the good results of irradiating choroidal metastases,
where it is sometimes possible to restore the vision in the affected eye. The irradiation of cerebral metastases is generally done post-operatively. If no operation is
done to relieve compression, steroids should be combined with irradiation to prevent
edema.

We have virtually given up injections of radioactive gold in the serous membranes because of the complications which ensue (symphyses).

Pleural and peritoneal effusions which contain no neoplastic cells may often be
dried up for a long period by oral steroid therapy at a moderate dose (25—30 µg
of prednisone per 24 h) combined with diuretics and a low-sodium diet. If this fails,
or if neoplastic cells are found, evacuation followed by injections into the serous
membrane of an antimitotic drug (a mustard of the Degranol type, for instance) are
indicated and may induce a more or less prolonged drying up of the effusion.

Hypophysectomy is the operation to be considered if all the preceding treatments have failed to give results. Its major indications are bone metastases, but it
may be justified in all other localizations, with the exception of visceral, cerebral
and, in particular, hepatic lesions.

To sum up: despite the diversity of the situations which confront him, the doctor's action to counteract the many forms of cancer assembled under Category C is

essentially on two planes: first, to slow down the development of the disease by treatments having a general field of action, such as hormone therapy; then to attempt by all available means—radiation, medication and, exceptionally, surgery—not simply to prolong life but to give the patients the best possible quality of physical and psychological comfort.

E. Treatment of Recurrences

By recurrences we mean all neoplastic lesions occurring in the regional sector: breast, chest wall, lymph-node areas, axillary, mammary and supraclavicular. It may well be that all these regions had already been treated at the time of the first treatment, or it may be that some were not, the extent of the first treatment differing from one patient to another.

Taking this fact into account, we can distinguish 3 main groups of recurrences:

a) recurrences in a region which has never been treated;

b) recurrences in a region which was not completely treated, that is to say, on which all the therapeutic resources were not exhausted; for example, a breast treated surgically but not radiologically;

c) recurrences in a region on which all therapeutic resources have already been used.

The therapeutic indications are fairly easy to establish in the first two cases, since there are still one or more ways of treating the disease which have not previously been used. The third group, on the other hand, often sets very difficult problems whose solution taxes the physician's ingenuity to the limit.

Whatever the conditions of their appearance, recurrences are a sign that the disease is still progressing and bear witness to its developing character. Treatments having a general action, capable of modifying this tendency, always deserve to be employed; castration in younger women and estrogen therapy in older women are justified as soon as the relapse is observed. Hypophysectomy, too, may also be considered for lesions which nothing else can check.

Recurrences seen in the breast following partial mammary interventions logically lead to an extension of surgery in the form of a simple or radial mastectomy. Recurrences in the chest wall after mastectomy or in the lymph nodes, when they are isolated and not numerous, may be removed surgically; but in our opinion the operation ought to be supplemented by radiotherapy. When there are too many to be dealt with by surgical means, radiation may sterilize them or at least stabilize them. If this is the first time radiation has been used, the technique is exactly the same as that used post-operatively to decelerate the tendency of the disease to progress in the regional sector. In addition, we give superdoses of 1500—3000 rads on the remnants of the lesions.

When radiotherapy has already been used in the zone where the relapse occurs, it is often possible to continue with it, either alone or after operation, but on limited fields in order to avoid post-radiotherapeutic complications. A very useful treatment here is interstitial radiotherapy by means of radioactive grains or threads, as it allows selective irradiation without doing too much damage to the normal tissues. However, cutaneous radionecroses are not unusual in such cases.

Relapses of the internal mammary lymph nodes are in a class by themselves. They appear in the form of more or less prominent parasternal tumefactions which can be homo- or contralateral to the lesion. Radiotherapy is usually effective at doses of 4000—6000 rads.

Finally, recurrences are always susceptible to forms of therapy which have not been used previously. It is true that it is possible to carry out successive excisions, or repeated irradiations at moderate doses. But their efficacy falls off rapidly and with radiation the risk of accidents increases fast. It is thus possible that the surgeon may act as second string in support of radiotherapy. Conversely, radiotherapy is frequently called upon where surgery has failed. In any case, hormone therapy should always form part of the treatment of recurrences.

1. False Recurrences

There are two diagnostic errors which can have serious consequences. The first consists in thinking that when edema of the arm is seen, this is necessarily a sign of recurrence. In the great majority of cases it is connected with more or less delayed regional modifications of the circulation if surgery or radiotherapy has been applied earlier. To apply more radiotherapy in this case would be extremely likely to make the situation worse, whereas steroid therapy, massage and patience may well bring relief to the patient.

The second error is to attribute to a recurrence symptoms which could be due to a somewhat delayed radio-lesion, whether cutaneous, nervous (plexus brachialis) or pulmonary. It is important to make sure of the true nature of these troubles because, here too, further radiotherapy would be disastrous. Steroid therapy can again help to alleviate the symptoms.

2. Treatment of Distant Metastases

The treatment of distant metastases seen at the time of the first treatment has already been described under Category C (b). What was said there applies equally to metastases occurring after an interval of time which may sometimes be very long.

Radiotherapy is really justified only when there are highly localized metastatic lesions, particularly bone and cutaneous metastases. In the case of extended metastases, it can, however, be very valuable in relieving painful foci in the bone.

As soon as the metastatic lesions under consideration reach a certain extension, it is obvious that treatments on a local scale (surgery or radiation) are superseded. This is when hormone therapy and chemotherapy must be brought into play.

Treatment by male hormones has enjoyed quite a vogue. It is certain that one quarter or one third of patients can benefit by it. Regressions of lesions can last for several months, and the anabolizing effect of these hormones is also useful in undernourished patients. Classically, the major indication for androgen therapy is in premenopausal patients; in fact, it seems to be almost as effective in older women. Bone metastases seem the most likely to yield to this form of treatment. On the whole, however, the treatment protocols at the Institut Gustave-Roussy do not include many male hormone treatments for the reasons we have already explained.

We do not, however, direct these criticisms at the non-virilizing androgens (derivatives of 19-nortestosterone) which are virtually inactive in relation to the cancer, but which may usefully contribute towards the restoration of the patient's protein capital.

Estrogens are useful over the age of 55. Lesions of the skin and soft tissues are most likely to respond to them.

Progesterone, or rather the combination estrogen/progestogen, may also for a time inhibit the evolution of cutaneous lesions.

Steroid therapy is an equally valuable weapon. At low doses (less than 50 mg of cortisone or 30 mg prednisone), it can effect useful analgesias in painful bone metastases. At the same doses, combined with diuretics and antimitotic injections into the serous membranes, it can dry up pleural and· peritoneal effusions. At very large doses (150 mg cortisone or 75 mg prednisone), it can effect what is almost a physiological adrenalectomy. We are not convinced that this method should be recommended.

Note that cortisone does not deserve the mistrust it sometimes excites when bone metastases are in question. The osteoporosis of Cushing's disease need not be feared when a hormone is to be administered for only a few months; moreover, it is probable that the osteoporotic action of the steroid is compensated by the slowing down of ACTH production, which controls the estrogen secretion of the adrenals.

Finally, hypophysectomy is a valuable endocrine surgical action when done in full awareness of its effects. Bone metastases, and secondarily pulmonary-pleural or cutaneous metastases, are the best indications for this operation, which, however, must be reserved for forms of the disease with a low development potential. Strong indicative value is attributed to the free period between mastectomy and the appearance of the first metastasis. In practice, hypophysectomy should not be done if this interval is less than 18 months. British authors [21, 23, 25] have also shown an interest in the urinary excretion of androgens: patients producing a daily rate of androsterone and etiocholanolone of more than 1.5 g are those who react best to these operations.

Table 34. *Hypophysiolysis — results of treatment in 200 cases*

Localization	No. of patients	No. of objective successes
Bone metastases	164	78
Nodular cutaneous metastases	30	8
Lymphangic cutaneous metastases	16	—
Pleural metastases	19	4
Pulmonary metastases	15	3
Lymphedematous swelling of arm	14	3
Active inflammation of breast	9	2
Hepatic metastases	6	—
Cerebral metastases	5	1
Peritoneal metastases	3	—
Choroid metastases	2	1

Note: This table refers to 200 patients but, as some of them presented with several localizations, the results are given under each heading. The action of hypophysiolysis may vary according to localization.

With the woman who is virtually past the menopause, hypophysectomy is done at the start. With the premenopausal woman, castration is the first endocrine treatment to be considered.

Only after the action of castration has been exhausted is hypophysectomy decided upon. As we have seen, the Institut Gustave-Roussy endorses hypophysiolysis by yttrium-90 implantation within the pituitary body; done by an experienced team and after strict selection, this gives remission of the lesions in 50% of cases.

Table 34 summarizes the results observed in the first 200 patients who benefited from hypophysiolysis.

It is as a rule only after the failure of hormone therapy that we resort to chemotherapy, according to the formulas stated earlier under Category C. Lesions of the soft tissues are most often influenced by it, but such remissions seldom last more than a few months. Moreover, it cannot be carried out effectively unless the patient's blood picture remains satisfactory.

3. Special Cases

Discharges From the Nipple

Non-bloody discharges without mammary tumor. After a cytological study of the liquid and mammography, with and without preparation, patients are mainly kept under observation where these examinations are negative. If either the cytology or the radiograph give reason to suspect trouble, they are entrusted to the surgeon who operates under the safeguard of frozen-section histology. The procedure is:

resection of the milk ducts if the microscopic examination is negative;

simple mastectomy if an intraductal epithelioma is suspected;

therapeutic program according to the corresponding category if an infiltrating carcinoma is found.

Bloody Discharges

Without mammary tumor—treatment is again decided by a frozen-section histological examination;

resection of the milk ducts, if negative;

simple mastectomy, if intraductal carcinoma is suspected;

with mammary tumor—in these cases, the discharge from the nipple is, so to speak, an additional phenomenon, and the tumor is classified like any other according to its extension and given the appropriate treatment. The microscopic examination indicates typical simple mastectomy if there is an intraductal epithelioma, and extended mastectomy according to the normal protocol once the carcinoma has gone beyond the bounds of the milk duct.

Paget's Disease

This can be apparently isolated or associated with a mammary tumor.

Paget's disease on its own. A mastectomy must be carried out in any case but it is also essential in the course of the operation to make an immediate microscopic examination of the epidermis of the nipple, since the deep tumor is often discovered only on detailed dissection of the fixed specimen; if the carcinoma is outside the ducts, the operation should be extended to radical mastectomy with internal mammary dissection.

Paget's disease with mammary tumor. Here the tumor has prime importance and, as with any other tumor, its extension will determine the choice of treatment.

Sarcomas of the Breast

As these lesions are not very sensitive to radiation, their treatment is basically surgical and consists in simple mastectomy with ablation of the underlying structures as required. If surgery seems inadequate, it may be supplemented by radiotherapy of the suspect scar region, up to the maximum doses of 6000 or 7000 rads according to the size of the volume treated.

Reticulosarcomas, lymphosarcomas, Hodgkin's disease, in all of which it is exceptional for the mammary localizations to be primary, obviously require treating according to the specific therapy for these diseases: regional radiotherapy at moderate doses (3500 rads) and chemotherapy.

Whenever the tissue of the mammary gland is not the point of departure of the lesion, hormone therapy does not come into question.

Breast Cancer in Men

Such cancers are classified by the same UICC system and fall into the same therapeutic categories.

The treatment protocol is identified for each group as regards surgery and radiotherapy, although it is different at the hormonal level. Castration, which should in theory be recommended, is simply not accepted, and we have given up suggesting it, even in advanced cases.

On the other hand, estrogen is systematically prescribed for men over 60 years of age with developed (Categories B and C) or developing cancers (PEV).

F. Cancer during Pregnancy

The association of breast cancer with pregnancy is well known to have a very unfavorable prognosis [46]. Indeed, the simultaneous presence or possibly the sequence of a mammary tumor and pregnancy poses a certain number of often very complex problems.

First, we must picture the various situations as they confront the clinician, bearing in mind that in every case technical and ethical problems are inextricably linked. After that, we shall group the cases, somewhat arbitrarily, under three headings.

Group A represents what we will call the "technical" situations.

Situation 1: when breast cancer or pregnancy occur together, should termination of pregnancy be considered or not? In other words, is termination of pregnancy thought beneficial with regard to the development of the cancer, hence will it benefit the mother in future?

Situation 2: should anti-cancer treatment, if considered to be indispensable, be regarded as exerting a dangerous influence on the fetus and hence as being on its own account an indication for abortion, even supposing that the existence of a breast tumor did not in itself justify termination of pregnancy?

In the final analysis these questions will be most easily answered if judgement is based on the essential points, on criteria which are as precise and objective as possible.

Group B includes cases of breast cancer which have been treated previously; here the essential problem is to know whether to advise against any subsequent pregnancy, either for a limited period or once and for all.

Group C, finally, includes the cases where the question that arises is whether to continue with breast feeding or whether to wean the baby.

Problems of Group A

First, a few facts:

1. there is no doubt at all that pregnancy greatly aggravates cancer of the breast;

2. this aggravation seems generally to be associated with the developing forms. It is possible that, to some extent, at least, the diagnosis will have been made rather late, owing to the very great modifications which take place in this organ during gestation. This was the case with two of our patients on whom, at other hospitals, a most ill-timed incision of the tumor was made after an abscess had been diagnosed;

3. N− cancers, which are the less severe forms (without lymph-node invasion) behave like ordinary cancers where pregnancy is not present;

4. on the other hand, the severe forms, N+ or developing, are made much more serious by their association with pregnancy;

5. pregnancy was terminated in 7 cases. These are too few to enable conclusions to be drawn on the basis of this experience, but it was of no obvious benefit to the patients, who were selected in the absence of any particular indication.

We must, however, stress the difficulty of such a study and the dangers inherent in reaching a premature conclusion on the basis of results obtained from too small a number of patients.

This condition, indeed, is so rare as to limit the extent of the studies devoted to it. On a strictly medical plane, there is thus no argument supported by objective results which allows us to assert that termination of pregnancy is capable of modifying the course of breast cancer. Some authors have even wondered whether abortion might not carry the risk of worsening it. We do not at present seem to have at our disposal any facts which support such a hypothesis. Indeed, the inadequacy of the data is such that we cannot reach any conclusion regarding abortion and whether it is or is not beneficial in cases of breast cancer. There is thus no question of recommending it in any systematic manner and in the hope of improving the chance of survival so long as we have no definite evidence one way or the other.

Now we must consider to what extent the actual treatment—surgery, irradiation, chemotherapy—may *endanger the fetus.*

The general opinion is that surgery does not constitute a danger. Moreover, when the treatment protocol for breast cancer comprises surgery alone, it is because stable and not very extensive forms are involved. The treatment may be carried out without regard to the existence of pregnancy, but with the normal precautions. On the other hand, extensive or developing forms of cancer require irradiation as the first treatment. We must then consider what will be the dose received by the fetus and whether this dose constitutes a danger.

The risks to the embryo and fetus have been the subject of a report presented to the "Commission de l'Enfance et de la Maternité" of the "Ministère de la Santé Publique" at its meeting of 29th June, 1962. According to this report, it appears that a dose of more than 20 rads in the early months and 50 rads in the later months could be dangerous for the embryo or fetus. According to the techniques of irradiation employed, the dose received by the fetus may vary and must be carefully calculated for every case.

Table 35. *Dose received by the fetus during irradiation of a mammary field 17 cm high*

Distance between fetus and base of irradiation field (cm)	Dose received by the fetus when dose received by tumor is (rads)		
	4500	7500	9000
5	180	300	360
10	90	150	180
15	55	90	110
20	30	50	60
25	20	33	40

As an example, we quote the telecobalt technique used at the Institut Gustave-Roussy, where the dose administered at the level of the breast and the lymph-node areas is between 4500 and 9000 rads. We must therefore calculate that in the first months of pregnancy the fetus would receive a total dose (at the IGR) of about 50 rads, which would certainly involve a teratogenic risk. During the final months of pregnancy, the risk of teratogeny will virtually have disappeared, but the uterus is now bigger und the doses received by the fetus will fall within the range of 40—180 rads. There is thus a not inconsiderable risk of inducing leukemia or cancer.

As for chemotherapy, which is by definition cytotoxic, it would appear to be *a priori* highly teratogenic. Therefore it would be only prudent to refrain from using it at any stage of pregnancy.

Problems of Group B

Let us now consider the problems raised by the cases which fall into Group B. The patient has been treated and later becomes pregnant. If we base our arguments on work done on such patients, we can accept that there is not a very great risk of aggravating the disease, but that it is nevertheless desirable that pregnancy be avoided in the 2 or 3 years immediately following the conclusion of treatment. However, should a pregnancy occur, with no sign of any recurrence of the cancer, there is no reason to advise its termination. If, on the the other hand, there is some manifestation of cancer, treatment will depend on the clinical form this takes and will accordingly fall into one of the situations already considered under Group A.

Furthermore, if we assume that, particularly in N+ cases, it is better to avoid all risk of pregnancy for 2 or 3 years, then a mechanical method of contraception should be suggested to the patient, since the risk of hormonal contraception after treatment for breast cancer is still an unknown factor. This, of course, applies only in cases where castration has not been done, this being the normal supplementary treatment in the policy adopted at the Institut Gustave-Roussy for N+ and non-surgical forms.

Problems of Group C

Finally, we must mention the problems raised by the situations included under Group C. These concern a cancer which appears during lactation. Twelve of our patients fell into this category and, of these, five have survived for 5 years. Some even recommend maintaining the secretion of milk by mechanical means while switching the infant to artificial feeding.

These, therefore, are the various situations which can arise when cancer and pregnancy coincide. In order to resolve the resulting problems, the doctor must first, in consultation with those of his colleagues who are concerned, establish the precise extent of the risks of the cancer and the risk to the fetus. Only when these risks have been clearly defined can the doctor discuss them with the prospective parents.

He may set out two possibilities:

1. there is no medical indication for termination of pregnancy, since the form of the disease is of limited extension and not developing, hence a case for initial surgical treatment. This must be explained to the family, they must be reassured and the pregnancy allowed to run its course;

2. the treatment which is judged to be indispensable offers such grave risks to the fetus that it is necessary to discuss the indications for abortion. The parents are quite free to accept or reject it. But if they decide to reject it, the doctor then has to face a very delicate problem, which is to decide whether he is justified in modifying the treatment so as to ensure the maximum protection for the fetus.

To sum up, for us, the only acceptable indication for termination of pregnancy is the danger to the fetus from the proposed treatment.

In conclusion, apart from the very restricted situation which in our opinion justifies the discussion of abortion, there is no other indication for the termination of pregnancy during the development of breast cancer, but it is obvious that, even in such cases, the final decision as to whether to accept or reject the abortion recommended by the doctor in the only case where he considers it justified must rest with the mother, and will be conditioned by her religious beliefs, her desire for a child, and her family and social background. The doctor, in our opinion, must abide by strictly medical arguments; he must be neutral as regards all the other aspects of the problem.

IV. Results

We have explained the policy on which we base our treatment at the Institut Gustave-Roussy, the therapeutic indications themselves, and the team-work organization within which the treatments are planned. Now it is time to present the results we have obtained by carrying out this policy as faithfully as possible.

Table 36 groups the results under therapeutic categories, but it includes only the 916 patients for whom the protocol was followed exactly. For all cases treated, the tables in Appendices A and B should be consulted. Moreover, to enable others to compare our results with their own, we present as Appendices C, D and E a set of tables where our material is arranged according to the various possibilities of the T N M classification and some other criteria. This is a good example of the advantage of such a classification, since it allows results to be presented in a way which, while it emphasizes aspects of the problem as required, yet retains comparability with other methods of expression. The important thing is that the basic distribution, i. e. the contents of each category under T, N and M, should be published systematically.

Table 36. *Period 1954—1962 — Treatment of malignant breast tumors in 916 patients for whom the protocol was followed exactly*

		No. of cases with 5-yr follow-up	No. living after 5 yrs	Survival rate
A	N−	145	126	87%
	N+	254	174	68%
	total A	399	300	75%
A′	. . . .	60	30	50%
A+A′	. . . .	459	330	72%
B	. . . .	242	72	30%
C	chest wall fixation	35	5	14%
	distant metastases	180	17	9%
Total		916	424	46%

In Table 36, where the results are given under our therapeutic categories, we have made a special distinction between Category B and an intermediate category, A′, which is quite simply the category for patients who would have been placed in Category A had they not had a developing phase. We thought it necessary, for clarity of presentation and to facilitate subsequent comparison, to make this distinction in presenting the results. The reason is that, in places where the idea of the developing phase is not yet accepted, and where the existence of this condition is not regarded as a contraindication to surgery, it is quite evident that the category of surgical patients, although it may contain patients on whom we too would operate, should, if we wish to make a fair comparison, also include the patients who have a developing growth (PEV 1). This is why we have introduced this additional category.

Furthermore, within Category A, we have—since this is a subdivision which arises naturally along the way—distributed the cases according to the condition of the lymph nodes. Finally, for Category C, we thought it desirable to divide this, too, according to the two trends, since they lead to two rather different forms of treatment: there are C patients with regional predominance, and C patients with distant metastases.

A study of Table 36 will show that the Category A N— cases, who for this reason have received only surgical treatment without supplementary radiotherapy, have an 87% 5-year survival rate. Where there is invasion of the lymph nodes, i. e. Category A N+, and supplementary radiotherapy has been given, accompanied by castration if the patient was premenopausal or less than 2 years postmenopausal, the 5-year survival rate falls to 68%. Taking both parts of Category A together gives a survival rate of 75% for 330 patients.

We must stress that in Category A N—, where we had an 87% survival rate and hence a 13% failure rate, we did not observe among this group any new regional manifestations of the disease; all our failures were due to distant metastases. This confirms our original hypothesis (see p. 19) that true N— cases do not carry a risk of local recurrence, and it justifies our policy of withholding post-operative radiotherapy.

As regards Category A', we note that the 5-year survival rate is 50%; 60 cases were placed in this category, while 399 having the same extension but without the developing phase, were placed in Category A. This means that, in a hospital where the idea of the developing phase is not accepted, and where all the cases we include in Category A would be regarded as initially operable, they would have treated 459 patients by surgery. If we make allowance for this, we would have had a survival rate of 72%.

We also wish to emphasize the very clear difference between the three groups which might at first sight be considered similar:

	5-yr survival %
A N—	87
A N+	68
A PEV 1 (A')	50

Clearly, the severity of the A' forms is greater. We must once more stress that they were not classed as PEV 1 retrospectively; these patients were recognized and classed as "developing" at the time when the diagnosis was made at the beginning. From this time on they received a different form of treatment from the rest of Category A, one deploying all the resources at our disposal. We therefore think this proves conclusively that there is a special category here which deserves to be isolated.

As regards Category B, excluding Category A', the 5-year survival rate was 30%. Finally, Category C exhibits a slight difference according to whether the regional or distant form predominates, survival rates being 14 and 9% respectively.

Appendix A. *Five-year survival — All cases seen at the Institut Gustave-Roussy between 1954 and 1962. Cases given in brackets are those for which the protocol was followed (see table 36)*

Therapeutic categories		No. of cases	Surgery first								Miscellaneous
			Simple mastectomy with or without axillary dissection		Halsted or more		Radiotherapy before surgery		Radiotherapy only		
			No. of cases	Survival	No. of cases	Survival	No. of cases	Survival	No. of cases	Survival	
A	N−	159	9	67%	(145)	(87%)	4	75%	7	57%	1 alive
	N+	278	12	33%	(254)	(68%)	12	50%			
	NX	36	21	57%			4	75%			4 alive
	Total	473									
A′		62			2	DCD	(52)	(52%)	(8)	(37%)	
B		334	18	67%	74	61%	(152)	(39%)	(89)	(12%)	(1 alive)
C	chest wall fixation	37	2	50%			(6)	(17%)	(29)	(12%	
	distant metastases	180	(6)	(17%)	(5)	(80%)	(27)	(29%)	(134)	(4%)	(8) (12) %
Not classified		9	8 cases		87% survival				1 case deceased		
Lost to follow-up		79			48 cases		11		18	2	
Grand total		1174			599		268		286	16	

Appendix B. *Five-year survival — All cases seen 1954—1962*

		No. cases	Cases treated following protocol 5-yr survival	Cases treated differently from protocol 5-yr survival	All cases 5-yr survival
A	N−	159	87%	71%	79%
	N+	278	68%	42%	55%
	NX	36		64%	64%
	Total	473	75%	59%	66%
A′		62	50%	48%	49%
A+A′		535	72%	58%	60%
B		334	30%	32%	31%
C	regional	37	14%	35%	24%
	distant	180	9%		9%
Not classified		9		88%	88%
Lost to follow-up, classified as deceased		74			0%
Grand total		1174	46%	33%	40%

Appendix C. *Description of breast cancer population [a] from 1st January, 1954, to 30th June, 1962*

		All cases	1954—56 %	1957—59 %	1960—62 %
Metastases	no	956	87	80	85
	yes	184	13	20	15
Metastases excluded	T1	40	5	5	3
	T2	435	56	40	44
	T3	369	37	43	41
	T4	77	2	12	12
Size of tumor	≤ 5 cm	579	66	58	69
	> 6 cm	325	34	42	31
PEV	no	781	83	85	80
	yes	161	17	15	20
Axillary invasion (hist.)	N−	226	32	28	32
	N+	515	68	72	68
Internal mammary invasion (hist.)	N−	191	62	69	68
	N+	97	38	31	32
Total invasion (hist.)	Ax−IM−	55	19	17	22
	Ax+IM−	136	43	52	46
	Ax−IM+	4	3	1	—
	Ax+IM+	93	35	30	32
5-yr survival	alive	532	47	47	52
Incl. metastases	dead	563	53	53	48

[a] 79 cases are not included owing to lack of data.

Appendix D. *Survival as a function of clinical features (5-yr survival rate)*

		1954—1956			1957—1959			1960—1962		
		a.	d.	s%	a.	d.	s%	a.	d.	s%
Metastases	no	184	162	53	179	137	57	147	97	60
	yes	5	148	9	7	72	9	5	43	10
Metastases excluded	T1	14	2	88	12	2	86	7	—	100
	T2	121	66	65	96	30	76	75	27	74
	T3	41	83	33	60	66	48	54	43	56
	T4	1	6	14	3	35	8	5	26	16
Size of tumor	≦ 5 cm	141	72	66	126	51	71	108	49	69
	> 6 cm	36	76	32	44	78	36	32	46	41
PEV	no	167	119	58	167	101	62	128	57	69
	yes	17	42	29	11	33	25	16	34	32
Axillary invasion	N−	62	14	82	60	12	83	49	8	86
	N+	86	80	52	102	79	56	92	58	61
Internal mammary invasion	N−	43	19	69	55	15	79	41	9	82
	N+	14	25	36	15	14	56	17	8	68
Total invasion	Ax−IM−	14	4	78	15	2	88	12	1	92
	Ax+IM−	29	15	66	40	13	75	30	8	79
	Ax−IM+	3	—	100	1	—	—	—	—	—
	Ax+IM+	11	25	31	17	14	55	17	8	68

a. = alive; d. = dead; s% = % survival after 5 years.

Appendix E. *Five-yr survival 1954—1962 (classified by T, M, axillary nodes [histological invasion] and PEV)*

					No. of cases	a.	d.	s%
T1	M0	N−	PEV	no	18	17	1	94
				yes	—	—	—	—
		N+	PEV	no	11	9	2	82
				yes	—	—	—	—
		N unknown (no ax. diss.)			8	7	1	88
	M1				—	—	—	—
Total T1					37	33	4	89
T2	M0	N−	PEV	no	125	109	16	87
				yes	11	8	3	73
		N+	PEV	no	225	150	75	67
				yes	20	8	12	40
		N unknown (no ax. diss.)			34	17	17	50
	M1				25	4	21	16
Total T2					440	296	144	67
T3	M0	N−	PEV	no	37	28	9	36
				yes	4	4	—	—
				not sp.	1	—	1	—
		N+	PEV	no	143	75	68	52
				yes	51	18	33	35
				not sp.		3	1	—
		N unknown (no ax. diss.)			107	27	80	25
	M1				72	10	62	14
Total T3					419	165	254	39
T4	M0				76	9	67	12
	M1				74	3	71	4
Total T4					150	12	138	8
Grand total [a] of cases treated					1046	506	540	48

[a] 128 cases are not included for lack of data, including 74 lost to follow up.

References

1. HUGUENIN, R.: Quelques vérités premières (ou soi disant telles) sur le cancer, Vol. 1. Paris: Masson et Cie 1954.
2. DENOIX, P.: De la diversité des cancers du sein. Mém. Acad. Chir. 80, No. 19—20, 532—538 (1954).
3. — Monographie de l'Institut National d'Hygiène. No. 5, 257 (1954). De la diversité de certains cancers. A propos de 33.784 observations de cancers du sein, du col de l'utérus, de la langue, de la peau, du larynx, de l'oesophage et du rectum.
4. — GELLE, X.: Mode de décès des malades atteintes de tumeurs malignes du sein en fonction de l'envahissement microscopique du système lymphatique. Bull. Ass. franç. Cancer 42, No. 5, 548—555 (1955).
5. BERG, J. W.: The significance of axillary node levels in the study of breast carcinoma. Cancer 8, 776 (1955).
6. DENOIX, P.: A propos de l'envahissement lymphatique dans les cancers de la langue et du sein. Etude de 867 cas. Mém. Acad. Chir. 81, No. 8—9, 250—257 (1955). Bull. Ass. franç. Cancer 42, No. 2 (1955).
7. TALAIRACH, J., ABOULKER, J., TOURNOUX, P., DAVID, H.: Technique stéréotaxique de la chirurgie hypophysaire par voie nasale, suites opératoires, indications thérapeutiques. Neurochirurgie 2, 3—20 (1956).
8. FOULDS, L.: The natural history of cancer. J. chron. Dis. 8, 2—37 (1958).
9. VOGT-HOERNER, G., GERARD-MARCHANT, R.: Technique anatomo-pathologique de recherche et d'examen des ganglions lymphatiques. Bulletin du Cancer 45, 446—453 (1958).
10. DICSFALUZY, E., NOTTER, G., EDSMYR, F., WESTMAN, A.: Estrogen excretion in breast cancer patients before and after ovarian irradiation and oophorectomy. J. clin. Endocr. 19, 12—30, 1244 (1959).
11. HUGGINS, C.: On hormone dependent cancer. J. roy. Coll. Surg. (Edinb.) 4, 191—198 (1959).
12. JURET, P.: Éléments de pronostic biochimiques du cancer du sein. Bull. Ass. franç. Cancer 46, 535—562 (1959).
13. PICARD, J. D., DESPREZ-CURELY, J. P., ROUQUETTE, C.: Place de la mammographie parmi les éléments du pronostic des cancers du sein. Bull. Ass. franç. Cancer 46, 621—633 (1959).
14. ROUQUETTE, C., LELLOUCH, J., DENOIX, P.: Pronostic du cancer du sein en fonction d'un certain nombre de caractères cliniques. Bull. Ass. franç. Cancer 46, 599—620 (1959).
15. SCHWARTZ, D., JURET, P.: Valeur pronostique d'un groupe d'examens biologiques dans le cancer du sein métastatique. Bull. Ass. franç. Cancer 46, 563—569 (1959).
16. JURET, P.: A propos de l'action analgesique de l'hypophysectomie vis-à-vis des cancers métastatiques. Presse méd. 68, 1044—1046 (1960).
17. DENOIX, P.: Examens cliniques d'une malade s'inquiétant d'une tuméfaction mammaire. Gaz. méd. Fr. 67, 1205—1210 (1960).
18. SARRAZIN, D.: Altérations histopathologiques des tumeurs mammaires irradiées. A propos de 101 cas. Recherche de corrélations statistiques avec le pronostic. Mémoire pour le C.E.S. d'Electroradiologie. Paris 1960.
19. VOGT-HOERNER, G.: Propagations intramammaires dans les cancers du sein et rapports avec l'envahissement des ganglions lymphatiques axillaires. Bulletin du Cancer 7, No. 2, 279—290 (1960).
20. CONTESSO, G.: Etude histologique et comparative des caricnomes mammaires avant et après irradiation. Mémoire pour le C.E.S. d'Anatomie-Pathologique. Paris 1961.

21. DAO, L. Y., HUGGINS, C.: Bilateral adrenalectomy in the treatment of cancer of the breast. Arch. Surg. 71, 645—657 (1962).
22. DENOIX, P.: Importance des relations hôte-tumeur dans l'évolution des cancers humains. Rev. franç. Étud. clin. biol. 7, 241—245 (1962).
23. ATKINS, H.: A preoperative assessment of response to the operations of adrenalectomy and hypophysectomy. In: Symposium on the prognosis of malignant tumors of the breast, Vol. 1. Eds.: P. DENOIX and C. ROUQUETTE. Basel-New York: S. Karger 1963.
24. BLOOM, H. J. C.: The role of histological grading in the study of breast cancer. In: Symposium on the prognosis of malignant tumours of the breast. Paris 1962. Eds.: P. DENOIX and C. ROUQUETTE. Basel: S. Karger 1963.
25. HAYWARD, J. L., BULBROOK, R. D.: The relation between steroid hormone excretion and survival after mastectomy. In: Symposium on the prognosis of malignant tumors of the breast, Vol. 1. Eds.: P. DENOIX and C. ROUQUETTE. Basel-New York: S. Karger 1963.
26. LALANNE, C. M.: Taux d'accroissement et pronostic des tumeurs malignes du sein. In: Symposium on the prognosis of malignant tumours of the breast. Paris 11., 12. 13. juillet 1962. Eds.: P. DENOIX et C. ROUQUETTE. Basel: S. Karger 1963, p. 16—23.
27. PICARD, J. D.: Rôle de la mammographie dans le pronostic des tumeurs malignes du sein. L'aspect oedémateux malin. Discussion caractères cliniques et pronostic. In: Symposium on the prognosis of malignant tumours of breast. Paris 1962. Eds.: P. DENOIX et C. L. ROUQUETTE. Basel: S. Karger 1963, pp. 32—44.
28. VOGT-HOERNER, G.: Valeur pronostique de quelques critères anatomo-pathologiques dans les tumeurs malignes du sein. L'envahissement du mamelon. In: Symposium on the prognosis of malignant tumours of breast. Paris 1962. Eds.: P. DENOIX et C. ROUQUETTE. Basel: S. Karger 1963, pp. 45—50.
29. ROUQUETTE, C.: Envahissement ganglionnaire et pronostic des tumeurs malignes du sein. In: Symposium on the prognosis of malignant tumours of breast. Paris 1962. Eds.: P. DENOIX et C. ROUQUETTE. Basel: S. Karger 1963, pp. 77—84.
30. JURET, P.: Eléments de pronostic biochimique du cancer du sein: réaction inflammatoire et cholestérolèmie... discussion. In: Symposium on the prognosis of malignant tumours of breast. Paris 1962. Esd.: P. DENOIX et C. ROUQUETTE. Basel: S. Karger 1963, pp. 172—181.
31. VOGT-HOERNER, G., CONTESSO, G.: Localisation anatomique du premier ganglion axillaire métastatique du cancer du sein (à propos de 73 observations n'ayant qu'un seul ganglion axillaire envahi). J. Chir. (Paris) 86, No. 12, 37—42 (1963).
32. JURET, P., HAYEM, M., FLAISLER, A.: A propos de 150 implantations d'Yttrium radio-actif intra-hypophysaire dans le traitement du cancer du sein à un stade avancé. J. Chir. (Paris) 87, 409—433 (1964).
33. LALANNE, C. M., SARRAZIN, D., ASCARELLI, A., JUILLARD, G.: La télécobalthérapie à l'Institut Gustave-Roussy. IV. Tumori della mamella. Nunt. radiol. (Roma) 30, 1 (1964).
34. VOGT-HOERNER, G., LALANNE, C., JURET, P., LACOUR, J., HOURTOULE, F., ROUJEAU, J., ROUQETTE, C.: Survie à la cinquième année d'une série de 237 cancers du sein opérés d'emblée. Mém. Acad. Chir. 90, 653—659 (1964).
35. CONTESSO, G.: Contribution à l'étude du pronostic histologique des cancers du sein. Thèse Paris 1965.
36. DENOIX, P.: Le traitement des tumeurs en fonction de nos connaissances concernant le rôle de l'hôte. Rev. franç. Étud. clin. biol. 10, 583—586 (1965).
37. HAYEM, M., JURET, P.: A propos de cent cas d'abord de l'hypophyse par voie nasale dans le traitement de certains cancers hormono-sensibles. Ann. Oto-laryng. (Paris) 81, 547—566 (1965).
38. DENOIX, P., VOGT-HOERNER, G., LACOUR, J., HOURTOULE, F., LALANNE, C., ROUJEAU, J., JURET, P., ROUQUETTE, C.: De l'envahissement lymphatique dans les tumeurs malignes. Arch. Union Balk. 4, 425—436 (1966).
39. JURET, P.: Assessment of response at the Institut Gustave-Roussy. In: Clinical evaluation in breast cancer. Eds.: HAYWARD and BULBROOK. London: Acad. Press 1966, pp. 185—194.
40. — LALANNE, C. M., HENRY, R., HOURTOULE, F., FERMANIAN, J.: Valeur comparée de la castration chirurgicale et de la castration par les radiations d'après la mesure du taux des gonadotrophines urinaires. Rev. franç. Étud. clin. biol. 11, 176—182 (1966).
41. — Endocrine surgery in human cancers. Springfield (Ill.): Charles C Thomas 1966.

42. LALANNE, C. M., JURET, P., HOURTOULE, F., SARRAZIN, D., ROUQUETTE, C.: Essai de classification clinique TNM dans le cancer du sein. Int. J. Cancer 1, 613 (1966).

43. MACKAY, E. N., SELLERS, A. H.: A clinical trial of TNM staging of breast cancer 1960—1962. Medical Statistics Branch. Ontario-Dept. of Health Toronto. Int. J. Cancer 1, 515—524 (1966).

44. SARRAZIN, D., LALANNE, C. M.: La télécobalthérapie à doses elevées des cancers mammaires: évolution locale et séquelles. Ann. Radiol. No. 3—4, 377 (1966).

45. MACDONALD, I.: The natural history of mammary carcinoma. Amer. J. Surg. III, 435—442 (1966).

46. LACOUR, J., MOURALI, N., WEILER, J., DENOIX, P.: Cancer du sein et grossesse. A propos de 62 cas observés à l'IGR de 1949 à 1959. Rev. Prat. (Paris) XVII, No. 9, 1231—1239 (1967).

47. — HOURTOULE, F.: La place de la chirurgie dans le traitement des formes évolutives du cancer du sein. Mém. Acad. Chir. 93, 635—643 (1967).

48. LALANNE, C., JURET, P., HOURTOULE, F., SARRAZIN, D.: La castration dans le cancer du sein: chirurgie ou radiations? Vol. 6. Acta radiol. 4, 323 (1967).

49. VOGT-HOERNER, G., CONTESSO, G.: Répartition des ganglions axillaires métastatiques dans le cancer du sein. Mém. Acad. Chir. 93, 795—799 (1967).

50. SARRAZIN, D., LACOUR, J., JURET, P.: Protocole schématique de traitement des cancers du sein en phase évolutive. Protocole schématique de traitement des cancers du sein à l'IGR. Protocole schématique de traitement des cancers du sein métastatique. Rev. Prat. (Paris) XVIII, No. 25, octobre 1968, p. 3607—3615.

51. GENIN, J., MICHEL, G., LACOUR, J.: La chirurgie loco-régionale dans le traitement du cancer du sein. Rev. Prat. (Paris) XVIII, No. 25, octobre 1968, p. 3529.

52. JURET, P., HAYEM, M.: La chirurgie endocrinienne majeure. Rev. Prat. (Paris) XVIII, No. 25, octobre 1968, p. 3585.

53. — La castration dans le traitement du cancer du sein, problèmes d'actualité. Rev. Prat. (Paris) XVIII, No. 25, octobre 1968, p. 3575.

54. — L'hormonothérapie médicamenteuse dans le traitement du cancer du sein. Rev. Prat. (Paris) XVIII, No. 25, octobre 1968, p. 3563.

55. BRULE, G., JURET, P.: La chimiothérapie des cancers du sein. Rev. Prat. (Paris) XVIII, No. 25, octobre 1968, p. 3551.

56. LEZER, J.: Bilan anatomopathologique à propos de 19 femmes hypophysectomisées par implantation de matériel radioactif pour cancer d'un stade avancé. Thèse, Paris 1968.

57. MAY-LEVIN, F.: Etude des réactions d'hypersensibilité retardée chez les sujets porteurs de tumeurs solides en fonction de l'invasion ganglionnaire. Extrait de «Corso superiore di aggiornamento in oncologia clinica». Milan, 3 juin 1968.

58. MOISY, M., EPOUSE, LE: Intérêts et méthodes des études pronostiques en cancérologie mammaire: applications du cancer du sein. Thèse, Paris 1968.

59. ROUQUETTE, C.: Résultats en fonction de la classification. Rev. Prat. (Paris) XVIII, No. 25, octobre 1968, p. 3639.

60. SARRAZIN, D.: La radiothérapie des cancers du sein. Rev. Prat. (Paris) XVIII, No. 25, octobre 1968, p. 3537.

61. VOGT-HOERNER, G., CONTESSO, G.: Ganglions interpectoraux et cancers du sein. Int. J. Cancer 3, 35—38 (1968).

62. MALAISE, E., DENOIX, P.: La cinétique de la croissance tumorale. Concours méd. 7, VI (91—23), 4863—4873 (1969).

63. JURET, P., HAYEM, M., ESTELIN, R., MARKOVITS, P., SARRAZIN, D., LALANNE, C., PIERQUIN, B.: L'implantation d'Yttrium 90 intra-hypophysaire dans le traitement des cancers du sein à un stade avancé. Bilan de 300 interventions. J. Radiol. 1969.

64. BLACHE, M.: Etude statistique à propos de 1103 cas d'autopsies de cancéreux pratiquées à l'Institut Gustave-Roussy de 1960 à 1966 (à paraitre).

In Production

In Preparation